Dying To
WIN

Dying To
WIN

The Athlete's Guide to Safe and Unsafe Drugs in Sports

Dr. Michael J. Asken, Ph.D.

ACROPOLIS BOOKS LTD.
WASHINGTON, D.C.

Authorization to photocopy items for internal or personal use, or the internal or personal use of specific clients, is granted by Acropolis Books Ltd., provided that the base fee of $1.00 per copy, plus $.10 per page is paid directly to Copyright Clearance Center, 27 Congress Street, Salem, MA 01970. For those organizations that have been granted a photocopy license by CCC, a separate system of payment has been arranged. The fee code for users of the Transactional Reporting Service is: "ISBN 0-87491-887-1/88 $1.00 + .10"

ACROPOLIS BOOKS LTD.
Alphons J. Hackl, Publisher
Colortone Building, 2400 17th St., N.W.
Washington, D.C. 20009

Attention: Schools and Corporations
ACROPOLIS books are available at quantity discounts with bulk purchase for educational, business, or sales promotional use.

For information, please write to: SPECIAL SALES DEPARTMENT, ACROPOLIS BOOKS LTD., 2400 17th St., N.W., Washington, D.C. 20009.

Are there Acropolis books you want but cannot find in your local stores?
You can get any Acropolis book title in print. Simply send title and retail price. Be sure to add postage and handling: $2.25 for orders up to $15.00; $3.00 for orders from $15.01 to $30.00; $3.75 for orders from $30.01 to $100.00; $4.50 for orders over $100.00. District of Columbia residents add applicable sales tax. Enclose check or money order only, no cash please, to:

ACROPOLIS BOOKS LTD.
2400 17th St., N.W.
WASHINGTON, D.C. 20009

Library of Congress Cataloging-in-Publication Data
Asken, Michael J.
  Dying to win.

  Includes index.
  1. Doping in sports. 2. Athletes—Drug use.
I. Title.
RC1230.A85 1988 613.8 88-14382
ISBN 0-87491-887-1 (pbk.)

Book design by Kathleen K. Cunningham

DEDICATION

To Kaitlyn, Tristen, and Kimberly, in the hope that their
unlimited potential in life and sport will be realized through
guidance, hard work, and their *natural* talents.

Preface

This book was written with considerable ambivalence. In some ways, it is a tragedy that the need exists for a book on drug abuse prevention for athletes. More positively, however, it represents acknowledgment of this problem and increasing attempts to intervene and prevent it. Most important, it represents an acknowledgment of concern for the overall health and well-being of athletes as people and individuals.

The purpose of this book is to educate athletes about the effects of drugs in sports, so that they can make an informed and intelligent choice about drug use. It is unique in that the book focuses specifically on drug use and abuse by athletes in sport. It does this because in many ways the world of the athlete is far different from that of the nonathlete.

The book begins by discussing the special reasons for athletes' becoming involved with drugs. An explanation of why drug use in sport is problematic both for the athlete and sport itself follows. An extensive description of the drugs abused by athletes comprises the middle portion of the book. Aspects such as the physical, behavorial, and psychological effects of drugs; sport performance effects of drugs; side effects and toxic effects of drugs, and sanctions for particular drugs are presented.

Following is a section of active exercises that athletes can "train in" or work through to help strengthen drug resistance skills. These can be done either individually or as a group or team effort. Included are such things as values clarification, assessment of coping skills, alternate strategies for enhancing performance without the use of drugs, and dealing with specific temptation situations.

Guidelines for the athlete with a medical problem that requires the use of medication for treatment are discussed in the following section.

Finally, on a more personal level, the book contains comments and views on the effects of drugs on sports and athletes from the experts themselves: athletes, sport psychologists, and others dedicated to having sport and athletes develop, succeed, and excel.

It is hoped the book will inform each individual athlete who reads it. It also can serve as the basis for a drug abuse prevention program for an entire team or sports program. Most of all, it is the goal of the book to help athletes reach a point where their decisions about drug use are made on an intelligent and informed basis, free of confusion and myth, devoid of undue pressure or coercion. It is believed that when drugs and sports are seen in this light, the conclusion will be reached that they are a bad combination and that skills to help avoid drug use in sport will have been strengthened. Finally, this book attempts to make a significant contribution to prevent athletes from dying to win.

This book was not the result of one individual's work; therefore, many thanks are due. First, recognition is extended to the various authors and researchers whose work is cited in the bibliography. Much of the material in this book is taken from these resources, and their contribution is acknowledged. It is also recommended that those readers with further interest should read these original works as well.

Special thanks is extended to Dr. Walter Severs, professor of neuroscience and pharmacology at the College of Medicine of the Pennsylvania State University, Milton S. Hershey Medical Center, Hershey, Pennsylvania. His help in reviewing and his valuable comments on the pharmacology portion of the book are greatly appreciated. Further appreciation is extended to Joan Price of the United States Olympic Committee's Drug Control Program for her expertise and the valuable information she provided. Vickie Gentzel and Connie Zies deserve thanks for their help in the early stages of the preparation of the manuscript.* Acknowledgment and gratitude go to John Hackl of Acropolis Books for his support, insight, and concern for athletes and sport, evidenced by his desire to publish this book. To Jerry May, I extend my thanks for writing the foreword to the book and perhaps, more important, for igniting my initial interest in sport psychology. Special gratitude goes to the sports professionals and others who have provided their comments and views in the last section of the book. They have done so because of their concern and commitment to sport and athletes. Finally, I owe untold appreciation to my wife, Renie, for her understanding during the time required to complete this book.

* And to Jill, Penny, Barb, and Carolyn for their help in the final stages. Special appreciation is expressed to Jean Bernard for her careful editing and insightful comments.

▌Foreword

In his book, *Dying to Win: An Athlete's Guide to Drugs and Sports,* Michael Asken has developed a practical, readable, and honest approach to understanding the prevention of drug abuse in sports. The overall philosophy is to educate the athlete to make informed decisions regarding drugs and sports in order to avoid use, or to try to help prevent increasing problems if one already has used drugs. Attention is given to drug abuse as it affects both the psychological health of the athlete and presumed performance enhancement.

The book has an excellent section that includes a self-test on the myths of drug abuse in sports. As a result of Dr. Asken's clinical expertise, experience, and research, he is well-versed on issues causing drug abuse among athletes—i.e., the pressure to win, the search for the optimal edge, societal role models, the drug culture generation, and the personal problems.

With understanding and care, Dr. Asken outlines a good case for not using drugs by providing information on health and myths, and by demonstrating the inconsistent results of many drugs. The book also presents a very practical way of saying no to drugs through exercises on values clarification and behavioral management programs. The importance of developing a support system as a further buffer against drugs in athletic performance is emphasized as well.

I believe athletes young and old, parents, coaches, psychologists, physicians, and trainers will find this book meaningful, realistic, and useful.

Jerry R. May, Ph.D.
Clinical Psychologist
Professor of Psychiatry and
   Behavioral Sciences
School of Medicine
University of Nevada at Reno

Chairman, Sports Psychology Committee
U.S. Olympic Committee

Team Psychologist, U.S. Alpine Ski Team

Contents

Contents

Introduction:
AN ATHLETE'S GUIDE TO DRUGS AND SPORTS

Introduction:

**AN ATHLETE'S GUIDE
TO DRUGS AND SPORTS** There is a
problem in sports today; how bad that problem is may be
difficult to say. Some people claim it's so widespread that it
is an epidemic. Some say this is an exaggeration. Some people
claim the problem could ruin sports forever. Some say this is
an exaggeration. Some people are very concerned about the
problem. Some say these people worry too much.

The problem is the use of drugs in sports—or rather the
abuse of drugs in sports. There is a place for drugs in sports—
drugs prescribed by and used under the guidance of a physician for good medical reasons. There is no place for the
abuse of drugs—using drugs without professional medical
advice, without medical need, beyond prescribed doses, for
other than intended purposes, for self-experimentation, on a
dare, or for the hell of it.

Who is right about how widespread the problem is doesn't
really matter. The problem does exist. Graham Reedy, former
team physician for the Oakland Raiders, said:

> There's no problem in society that doesn't
> exist in sports, so we're naive to think there's
> no drug problem in sports.[1]

The fact that drug abuse exists in sports, no matter how big
or small, means that it *can* affect *any* athlete. That is the

concern of those who care about sports. That is the concern of those who care about athletes.

That is the concern of this book—you the individual athlete. It is for you, the athlete, who may find yourself faced with the presence of drug use in your sport. You, the athlete, who may be thinking about using drugs. You, the athlete, who has tried drugs. You, the athlete, who may influence a teammate to use or avoid drugs.

To you, the athlete, who already knows you have a personal problem with drug use, this book is for you too. BUT it won't be enough. Read the book if you like—but get help. Better yet, get help first—then read the book. Go to your coach, teammate, team doctor, trainer, sport psychologist, teacher, guidance counselor, or parents. Go to someone now and begin to get help before the hard work and dreams of your sports career are rendered meaningless.

There are certain signs that suggest that an athlete may be using drugs. These signs include:

1 Difficulties with coordination

2 Muscular twitches

3 Red eyes

4 Pinpoint pupils

5 Listlessness, withdrawal

6 Decrease in motivation, "desire"

7 Careless personal appearance

8 Change in personality, behavior

9 Change in lifestyle, friends, routines

10 Change in health status[2]

If you recognize these signs in a friend, fellow athlete, or teammate, you should be concerned. If someone sees them in you and expresses caring and concern, recognize what these signs mean.

14

As an athlete you may feel special and, in fact, may be special, but you are not immune to addictive problems. Sport is not a safety zone. A recent article in *Sports Illustrated* said this about the drug problem:

> You want to learn a lesson, learn this: The Big Lie is over. Sports can't bury its head in the sand anymore; there are too many bodies buried there.[3]

Chapter One

Purpose and Philosophy:
WHERE THIS BOOK IS COMING FROM

Purpose and Philosophy

WHERE THIS BOOK IS COMING FROM

The problem of drug abuse in sports is a sensitive one. It raises strong feelings and opinions on both sides. Disagreements, if not outright arguments, can result. So what is the point of this book? What is it trying to do? Where is it coming from, philosophically?

The purpose of this book is to educate you about drugs in sports. It is to provide you with facts about the effect of drugs on sports performance and your health as an athlete and person. It is written to challenge you to think about what is important to you as an athlete and as a person, and how drug use can affect your priorities. Its purpose is to help you in your decision-making process about drug use in your athletic career; to help you make an informed, intelligent choice based on your own desires.

Is this book totally neutral and objective about drug use in sports? No. It would be dishonest to say that it was. It is very difficult for anybody to be totally neutral about drug issues. There is a bias here that drug use and abuse in sports is self-defeating and potentially very dangerous. However, this bias is not a hollow prejudice. It comes from examining the scientific data, the psychosocial research, and the past and present effect of drug abuse on athletes.

While this book does reflect a bias, it is not propaganda. As I said, the point of the book is to educate and challenge you. An honest attempt will be made to stick to the basic assumptions on which this book is written.

These assumptions include:

1 Drugs are available to athletes and probably always will be.

2 Each athlete must deal with drug questions and dilemmas on a personal level.

3 Drugs are not good or bad in themselves; how they are understood and used defines whether they are a beneficial tool or destructive force.

4 Decisions such as these about drug use are best made when you have valid and complete information.

5 There are alternative ways to achieve the results desired from drugs without using drugs.

6 There are some unique reasons why athletes (as differentiated from nonathletes) abuse and become addicted to drugs; there are also many common reasons as well.

7 Athletes are not immune to drug abuse and addiction.

8 The better you understand yourself, the easier your decisions about drug use will be.

9 Such decisions take time and effort.

10 Good decisions are facilitated by discussing issues with other people you understand, who understand you; who you care about, who care about you; and who have the knowledge and skills to help you.

To summarize, this book was written to:

1 Help you as an athlete to recognize the relationship of drugs and sports.

2 Help you as an athlete to develop an understanding and respect for all drugs and their use.

Purpose and Philosophy

3 Provide you as an athlete with factual and honest information about the legal, medical, social, and psychological aspects of drug use and sports.

4 Help you as an athlete to recognize there are alternatives to drug use.

5 Help you as an athlete to begin to develop skills to make your *own* choices about drug use.

6 Help you as an athlete to involve the people who are close to you and those to whom you are close in your decision.

This book will present information on drugs and sports honestly so that you can make your *own* decision about drug use. You will anyway. Making an educated decision is the smart way to do it.

Chapter Two

Beginnings:
GIVING THIS BOOK, AND YOURSELF, A CHANCE

Beginnings

**GIVING THIS BOOK,
AND YOURSELF, A CHANCE**   As was
said earlier, the topic of drug use in sports is a sensitive issue,
and one that has many strong feelings associated with it.
Because of that, it can be difficult to listen, hear, and understand things fully and objectively—to give what is being said
a fair break.

Some of you will agree with almost everything written here.
It will help confirm what you already think and believe. For
some of you, however, parts of this book may evoke a strong
response. Even though the information is factual, it may run
counter to what you hear, think, or believe. If this is the case,
you might have some of the responses listed in Table 2-1.

Whenever we're faced with information we don't like or don't
want to hear, our first reaction is to deny it. DENIAL means
that we reject its existence, its reality, its accuracy. Think about
the time you flunked a test or got a lower grade than you were
expecting. Wasn't your response something like:

"It can't be!"
"There must be a mistake here!"

You tried to deny it, but there it is. You went to check it out
with your teacher or professor only to find that no mistake was
made; the grade stood.

Your next response was probably that of ANGER at the
teacher:

1 DENIAL:
It's not true!

2 ANGER:
How can that happen to me? Why me!

3 BARGAIN:
Maybe it's partly true, but . . .

4 DEPRESSION:
It is true; I never admitted it before.

5 ACCEPTANCE:
I'm going to use this to help me and stop fighting it.

Typical Reactions to Information We Don't Want to Hear

Table 2-1

"How can he[1] do that to me?"
"Who does he think he is?"

You probably called the teacher some choice names, used some carefully selected adjectives, questioned the teacher's credentials, and in general, doubted his competence as a human being!

Your anger faded, but the grade remained. The usual next feeling and action is an attempt to BARGAIN. You decided that maybe you could talk your way into a better grade, make a deal:

"Maybe I can explain it was just a bad day."
"Maybe I can do a report to bring up the grade."
"Maybe I can stay every day and clean the erasers."
"Maybe I can promise never to take this class and bother the teacher again."

No deal. The grade remained. As the reality of being stuck with the grade sank in, so did DEPRESSION:

"What am I going to do now?"
"This can really be a bummer."
"Maybe I should have paid more attention."
"Maybe I am not making it—period."

The final—and healthy—response is beyond depression to ACCEPTANCE of the situation. The depression and the total experience can be used as a learning opportunity. Plans are made to remedy the situation as much as possible.

"I'll take the course over again next semester."

Plans are made to prevent a recurrence:

"I now know this course will require more study time."
"I'd better check my understanding of the material with someone who knows it well."

The whole situation is used to reflect upon and learn what it means for you as a person:

"I need to take academic pursuits more seriously."

"Not all subjects are a piece of cake to be passed with minimal work."

"Not doing well bothers me more than I thought."

"It feels good to know I have the ability to learn from my mistakes."

As you go through this book, try to be aware whether you are having feelings similar to those above. They can interfere with your learning.

Will you deny initially that substance abuse is a problem in sports in general? In your sport? On your team? For you?

If you recognize some problems as applying to you at some level, will you get angry and respond with:

"What do psychologists know anyway?"

"He probably never used drugs so he doesn't know."

"This is just typical grown-up garbage."

Maybe you won't get past the denial or anger; a lot of athletes don't. They are stuck there—not wanting to hear any more, not wanting to be challenged, not having to think or change or defend their position rationally. However, if you do, can you recognize when you are trying to bargain?

"Well, maybe there is some drug abuse—but maybe it isn't so bad."

"Well I *probably* won't get in trouble if I'm careful."

"Just using it once in a while couldn't really hurt."

When you come to realize that bargaining is a futile attempt to rationalize what you still do not want to totally accept, some depression may follow:

"It really could happen to me."

"It really does happen to others."

"I didn't know as much about it as I thought."

"I didn't think things through as well as I should have."

Don't get stuck at this point either. Use these negative feelings as a cue to continue your struggle to decide what you will do about drug abuse. Recognize that this progression of feelings is helpful and healthy. The fact that you have experienced them means that you probably are ready to make that informed choice, based on knowledge and independent thinking. You are ready to read, hear, listen, struggle, debate, share, and decide.

Chapter Three

A History of Drugs and Sports:

NOTHING NEW UNDER THE SUN

A History of Drugs and Sports

NOTHING NEW UNDER THE SUN

Athletes have always strived for excellence. The drive to be the best has always led to a search for "something special" to give an advantage. That special so-called edge has not always been new or more intense physical and skill training techniques. Often, it has been some chemical substance that the athlete hoped would give him superior ability.

Athletes have tried substances as quaint as a concoction of ass's hooves ground and boiled in oil with roses. They have also tried techniques as bizarre as the alleged insertion of air into the rectums of a European country's team's swimmers for added buoyancy at the 1976 Montreal Olympics. Neither of these approaches had an obvious effect on improving performance.

The ancient Greek physician Galen reported that athletes of the third century B.C. used stimulants. Herbs and mushrooms are reported to have been used to enhance performance by the Greek Olympians. Aztec athletes used a cactus-based stimulant resembling strychnine.

In the mid and late nineteenth century, boxers used a brandy and cocaine mixture as well as strychnine tablets. In 1965, Amsterdam Canal swimmers are said to have been caught using drugs containing caffeine. Other coca leaf preparations were used in the late nineteenth century. Vin Mariani, a mixture of wine and coca leaf abstract, known as "wine for athletes," was used by French cyclists.

In 1904, marathoner Thomas Hicks competed successfully in the Olympics. It took four physicians to revive him after his success, however, because he had taken brandy and strychnine. In the 1930s, powdered gelatin mixed in orange juice was believed to be a performance enhancer. Athletes have also used sugar cubes dipped in ether. Sprinters have tried using nitroglycerine to dilate the arteries of their hearts to improve performance.

Ludwig Prokop, professor of sports medicine and director of the Austrian Institute of Sports Medicine in Vienna, reported that his first encounter with substance abuse was in athletes at the Oslo Winter Olympic Games in 1952. There he found broken ampules and injection syringes in the locker room of speed skaters. He also reported seeing a classical case of strychnine cramp on the stage of the 1964 Weight Lifting World Championship. He writes of seeing the same evidence of drug abuse again in speed skaters at the 1964 Olympic Games at Innsbruck.

Drug use and abuse seems to have become particularly widespread during the 1960s. Stimulants were used and promoted widely among professional football teams during the decade. Much of this type of drug use apparently has declined because of the many problems associated with it. Anabolic steroids are said to have been part of the Olympics for the first time in 1964. Their use, which will be discussed in detail later, continues today amid much concern and controversy. Contemporary substance use and abuse continues today as evidenced by the drug trials of some of the Pittsburgh Pirates players or the death of University of Maryland basketball great Len Bias, who died of a cocaine overdose shortly after being signed by the Boston Celtics in the summer of 1986.

The presence of substance abuse among athletes, and in sports generally, does not mean that such use is the norm or that it has been legitimized. It also should not be interpreted as evidence that such substances guarantee improved performance. In fact, the variety of fad and fashion in substance use and abuse probably should suggest the opposite. If success is as simple as ingesting such a substance, why the constant search for even more?

What the presence of substance use and abuse in the history of sports says—and why this history is presented here—is that drugs have always existed in sports and, no doubt, always will. Therefore, athletes need to find out all they can about drugs so that they can make informed decisions about using or avoiding them.

Chapter Four

Drugs and Sports:
A MYTH AND REALITIES SELF-TEST

Drugs and Sports

A MYTHS AND REALITIES SELF-TEST

Many myths, misconceptions, half-truths, and just plain non-sense exist surrounding drug use and sports. Below are some typical beliefs about drug use and sports. Take a moment to see how well you can separate the myths from the realities. Circle T if you believe the statement is true or F if you believe the statement is false.

1   It is harder for athletes to become addicted   T   F
    to drugs than it is for nonathletes.

2   Almost all athletes are against drug testing   T   F
    as a way to monitor and control drug abuse
    in sports.

3   Alcohol is the least abused drug among ath-   T   F
    letes.

4   Female athletes have much less of a drug   T   F
    abuse problem than male athletes.

5   Athletes use drugs only to enhance perfor-   T   F
    mance and because of their strong desire to
    win and be the best.

6   Using drugs is an acceptable personal choice   T   F
    because abuse only hurts the person using
    drugs.

7   The superior health of athletes protects them   T   F
    from drug reactions and addiction.

8   Just as most teenagers use drugs, most ath-   T   F
     letes use drugs in some form.

9   All athletes who abuse drugs have emotional   T   F
     problems.

10   A good way to know if a drug works and how   T   F
     it will affect you is to ask another athlete who
     has tried it.

11   If using a drug is the only way to insure being   T   F
     the best, any athlete would use it.

12   Even though there may be danger involved   T   F
     in taking a drug, the risk could be worth it
     because an athlete's performance is guar-
     anteed to be enhanced by it.

13   Because of tough competition some sports   T   F
     "require" drugs to allow athletes to compete
     successfully against one another.

14   Athletes are almost always aware of the   T   F
     sanctions against drug use.

15   Substances that are banned by sport regu-
     lating organizations are found only in illegal
     street drugs.

The answer to all these statements is FALSE (see Table 4-1). None are true and the reasons for this will become clear as you read the rest of this book. If you got most of these answers right, you are off to a good start at making an independent decision about drug use in sport. If you didn't do well, don't worry, but do read the rest of this book carefully. It will provide enough information for you to have a realistic picture of drug use and abuse.

Table 4-1
Myths About Drug Use In Sport

It is harder for athletes to become addicted to drugs than it is for nonathletes.

Almost all athletes are against drug testing as a way to monitor and control drug abuse in sport.

Alcohol is the least abused drug among athletes.

Female athletes have much less of a drug abuse problem than male athletes.

Athletes use drugs only to enhance performance and because of their strong desire to win and be the best.

Using drugs is an acceptable personal choice because abuse only hurts the person using drugs.

The superior health of athletes protects them from drug reactions addiction.

Just as most teenagers use drugs, most athletes use drugs in some form.

All athletes who abuse drugs have emotional problems.

A good way to know if a drug works and how it will affect you is to ask another athlete who has tried it.

If using a drug is the only way to insure being the best, any athlete would use it.

Even though there may be danger involved in taking a drug, the risk could be worth it because an athlete's performance is guaranteed to be enhanced by it.

Some sports "require" drugs to allow athletes to compete successfully with one another.

Athletes are almost always aware of the sanctions against drug use.

Substances that are banned by sport-regulating organizations are found only in illegal street drugs.

Chapter Five

Drugs and Sports Part Two

ARE THEY REALLY A PROBLEM?

Drugs and Sports Part Two

ARE THEY REALLY A PROBLEM?

How do we really know how widespread drug use is among athletes? The fact is, we probably don't. It is very difficult to get an accurate picture of how many athletes use or abuse drugs for several reasons.

Few studies have looked at this question. Surveys and studies that do exist represent a limited number of athletes or a limited area of the country, and they may not be representative of all athletes in all sports. Finally, there is an understandable reluctance among athletes to admit to drug use. Researchers say that even when confidentiality and anonymity are assured, athletes hesitate to discuss the problem. The same is true for coaches, trainers, and even team physicians.

Nonetheless, some surveys and studies exist. While they are not perfect and are subject to the above limitations, they begin to give some picture of the situation. When data from different sources are consistent, more confidence can be placed in the accuracy of that data.

Drug use in general in the United States has been changing and increasing. For example, the National Institute of Drug Abuse reported that between 1962 and 1980, the number of Americans who tried marijuana rose from 4 percent to 58 percent. The number of adults age 18 to 25 who have experimented with such harder drugs as cocaine, heroin, hallucinogens, and inhalants rose from 3 percent to 33 percent.

The United States Department of Health and Human Services (HHS) reported changes in drug use between 1975 and 1980. According to the report, one-third of students have tried marijuana before entering high school. Cocaine use by young adults increased by 40 percent during that same time period. One trend that was seen and described as most disturbing was a shift to the use of more than one drug.

What about athletes? A recent study was conducted by the Minnesota Department of Public Welfare. This research included 3,000 ninth through twelfth grade students involved in sports as intramural participants, interscholastic athletes, trainers, or cheerleaders. Approximately one-third of the students had admitted to using beer or wine at least once a week, the students revealed. Approximately half said they had tried marijuana. One out of five of the study participants reported using marijuana weekly.

The use of most other drugs was found to be comparable to the general student body. However, amphetamine use by athletic participants was three times greater than that of nonparticipants.

Recent data from the Maine Sports Initiative for Coaches in Alcohol and Drug Prevention indicated that perhaps 60 to 80 percent of all high school athletes use alcohol or other drugs during the sports season. Weekly use was found in 10 percent of the athletes. Overall, athletes were found to use drugs at the same rate as nonathletes.

An example of a small but potentially helpful study was done* in one area of Pennsylvania. Coaches from 15 high schools in a five-county area responded to a question about drug/alcohol abuse as part of a questionnaire on sport psychology. Drug use (alcohol was not separated out) among athletes ranged from 1 to 30 percent with an average of 11.8 percent of athletes having a problem as reported by their coaches. Further, although nine of the 15 schools reported that their athletes participated in school-wide drug education programs, no school or athletic program had a specific plan for drug abuse prevention among athletes.

Some studies have involved both high school and college athletes. One such study found alcohol to be the drug most

*By the author.

46   Drugs and Sports, Part Two

often used by college athletes. Approximately 65 percent of athletes said they used alcohol regularly, which was similar to use reported by nonathletes. Also in this study, 20 percent of athletes admitted marijuana use, 16 percent smokeless tobacco use, and 7 percent cocaine use.

A study of Canadian athletes found similar results. Alcohol use was reported by 50 percent of the athletes, and for marijuana use, 23 percent answered positively. Use of stimulants was admitted by 10 percent of the athletes, but 20 percent said they would consider using them. Four percent of the athletes admitted using cocaine.

Drug use and abuse by professional athletes also is difficult to assess exactly. Newspaper headlines and lead stories on sports pages attest to the presence of the problem, but may distort its seriousness. Some data do exist, however. For example, the National Basketball Association established a toll-free, 24-hour drug counseling telephone line. In 1981, it was reported that 42 of the players in the league used it.

One well-known NFL coach recently reported that $60,000 and $25,000 were spent respectively by the team trying to help two of its football players with their drug problems. He further stated that during his years as a head coach, 20 to 30 players had been asked to leave because of drug problems.

For a long time it was believed that drug use was minimal among athletes and even less among female athletes. We now know this is not true, and there now is evidence that sex-based differences in drug abuse among athletes are disappearing. A survey of Big Ten Conference women's sports found that one in four coaches were concerned that their teams engaged in excessive social use of alcohol. Among high school coaches in women's sports, 14 percent said that they had helped female athletes seek professional help. It has been reported that two-thirds of college trainers believed their female athletes used amphetamines and cocaine to stay up for games and practice and to prevent emotional lows. Marijuana reportedly also is used to relax.

The few studies conducted, as well as anecdotal evidence, seem to show that drug use and abuse happens among athletes at many levels of competition. Several observations about athletes and drug use seem to emerge. First, not *all* athletes use drugs for performance enhancement or recreation. Second, drugs are not used for performance enhancement reasons alone. Third, drug abuse among athletes shares some similarities with drug use among nonathletes. Fourth, while there are similarities in the way athletes use drugs, there are some differences as well. Fifth, because of the difficulty of collecting accurate data on athletes' use of drugs, current figures probably underestimate the problem.

Chapter Six

Why Athletes Do Drugs:
PROBLEMS, PRESSURES, PAIN, AND PLEASURE

Why Athletes Do Drugs:

PROBLEMS, PRESSURES, PAIN, AND PLEASURE Athletes do drugs for many different reasons (see Table 6-1). While the decision to use drugs is always a personal one, many factors influence this decision. Many reasons athletes use drugs are the same as those for nonathletes. This is especially true for the athlete who uses drugs for so-called recreational purposes—just for the experience or anticipated enjoyment.

Athletes have another category of reasons for using drugs, one that is related to their sport competition. Athletes may use drugs because they believe the drugs will enhance or improve performance. Within these two broad categories of reasons for drug use—recreation and performance enhancement, there are many specific reasons. It is worthwhile to look at some of them.

THE PRESSURE TO WIN

The will to win is basic to any competitive athlete. The motivation to be number one certainly can help to bring out the best in an athlete. However, if this motivation gets out of hand, it can also bring out the worst, including resorting to drug use. Being a star athlete brings rewards—social and financial—in our society. Winners are respected, if not idolized. The desire to gain these rewards can be so great for an athlete that he

1 The pressure to win

2 The search for the "special edge"

3 Social acceptance of drug use and abuse

4 The drug culture and sports training

5 Pain and the misuse of sports science and sports training

6 Peer pressure

7 Media pressure

8 Recreation and experimentation

9 Personal problems

10 Enablers

Why Athletes Use Drugs
Table 6-1

will do just about anything to help his effort—including taking drugs.

Often the pressure to do drugs is found in athletes who are good, even very good, but just may not be the best. Knowing this, but still wanting the glory, they turn to chemical aids to supplement the missing talent or drive. The inability to accept competitive reality is a problem.

Being among the best produces its unique pressures too, most notably the need to remain the best. The expectations of oneself and others, especially when they are achieved, can be even harder to maintain. To help maintain achievements, or to ease the pain of not being able to sustain them, athletes often turn to drugs.

The pressure of winning does not come solely from within the athlete. Parents and friends have expectations, teams and schools have expectations, districts and states have expectations. All of these expectations lead to incredible pressure on the athletes. Consider the pressures at the elite level, where national attention is focused on the athlete. Imagine the pressure of representing the entire country in the Olympic games.

It is no wonder that some athletes turn to drugs to help them cope with such pressures. But not all athletes do. Flexibility in dealing with stresses, healthy coping mechanisms, genuine support, and clear values and priorities help other athletes handle such pressures without a chemical crutch.

THE SEARCH FOR THE "SPECIAL EDGE"

The desire for the competitive edge is closely related to the desire and pressure to win. Pressures from within and without keep athletes looking for the magic that will allow them to attain or hang on to the number one ranking.

Athletes hope for many things from drugs as performance enhancers. They seek an increase in strength and endurance, a delay in the onset of fatigue, and an increase in their ability to concentrate and tolerate pain. Whether drugs can actually deliver these effects and whether they can do so without harming the athlete are issues that will be discussed later.

SOCIAL ACCEPTANCE OF DRUG USE AND ABUSE

Because the use of drugs is so widespread, you certainly don't need to be an athlete to learn about it. Certain medications prescribed by physicians are very useful drugs. But people often take more than they are told. Many years ago, the Rolling Stones, in "Mother's Little Helper," warned about the abuse the valium: "And if you take more of those, you will get an overdose. . ."

In addition to prescription medications, over-the-counter drugs are almost limitless. A trip to any drugstore will reveal an amazing array of substances—medications to ease pain, to stimulate weight loss or gain, to induce or prevent sleep, and so on. Drugs like alcohol are used on social occasions or to self-medicate or relax after a difficult day.

Society even tells us that it's okay to use certain substances to "enhance performance." Though not usually thought of as performance enhancing in the athletic sense, a "pick-me-up" often is sought and obtained from coffee, tea, cola drinks, and the like because of their caffeine content. And, although not generally considered drug abuse, consuming 16 cups of coffee a day certainly can be considered caffeine abuse and can cause side effects (and withdrawal symptoms when consumption is cut back). Whether to deal with stress, relax, perk up, handle pain, or change behavior, many people turn to a physician, pharmacy, or vending machine. And, perhaps, too freely.

Society often lays the groundwork for drug use by the athlete; it certainly may do little to discourage such use. The athlete finds himself a member of two communities, the athletic and the social, both of which strongly influence the use of drugs.

THE DRUG CULTURE GENERATION

As mentioned above, society has always had a need for drugs. In addition, some people today feel that athletes reflect the even more flexible and liberal attitudes about drug use in recent years. According to Professor Harry Edwards of the University of California, 30 years ago if anyone abused drugs, he clearly knew it was wrong; acceptable and unacceptable were much more clear. In the 1960s and 1970s, however, there was much

Why Athletes Do Drugs

experimentation with drug use and attitudes were more liberal. It has been said that current athletes (like other young Americans) are the "first wave of the drug culture generation."

Today's athletes are growing up when right and wrong about drugs is much less clear. They may encounter more of the attitude that there is nothing wrong with using drugs, for whatever purpose. Therefore, not only is there the subtle modeling of drug use in society, there may be active encouragement as well. Athletes must be sure that those who talk about the benefits of drug use really know what they are talking about.

PAIN AND GAIN: MISUSE OF SPORTS SCIENCE AND SPORTS TRAINING

The goal of sports training is to help athletes develop their *natural* abilities to their highest potential. However, sometimes too much enthusiasm in helping the athlete can lead to the misuse of drugs and medications.

In searching for improved techniques, sports scientists, too, can look to chemical substance enhancers. Some people question whether it is philosophically and ethically sound for sports scientists even to consider researching drugs as potential performance enhancers. Whatever one may think about it, such research occurs. Anabolic steroids are said to have been introduced to athletic training by a physician who used them on himself.

Aside from the issue of whether drugs should be researched at all for sport competition purposes, the task of sports science is to evaluate whether techniques and approaches (or drugs) do affect performance and whether they do so safely. Unfortunately, because of the pressures to win and produce, a new approach or drug can be promoted before all the research evidence is in. And it is usually the information on the risks of the drug to the athlete that comes last. Athletes may be over-eager to try a new approach (or drug) and start using it before they get all the information on it. This is an uninformed and dangerous thing to do.

Sports medicine physicians also may find themselves in difficult situations in terms of drug use. While their first task is to insure the overall health of the athlete, they are often under great pressure to make the athlete able to play. For playoffs or championship meets, some physicians may give in to pressure to fix an injured athlete so that he can compete. Meaning well, they will prescribe medication in situations where they normally would not do so. Rather than using rest, therapy, and time, the doctor may prescribe something to get the athlete over the hump.

Athletes who are determined to compete may pressure their doctors into giving them drugs to combat the pain. Giving in to such pressure too frequently can become a problem for a physician. In addition, the athlete may find that the drug has worked well and may decide to use it on a regular basis. He may even decide that it would be easier to use the drug and continue playing rather than go through a full rehabilitation process.

The athlete may fail to realize the long-term danger of doing this. Any small pain or discomfort may prompt an athlete to start using a drug. Such use can quickly become a problem, and may lead to addiction. The athlete will seek the drug from the sports medicine physician or, if it is refused, from any other available source.

The coaching and training staff can also be instrumental in an athlete's drug use. Although the overall health of the athlete should be the concern of the coach and training staff, this is not always the case. Some staffs may place so much emphasis on winning and so much pressure on athletes that the athlete starts to look to drugs for help. In rare instances, the staff actually may encourage the athlete to use something for a special situation to enhance performance, or worse may even provide the drug.

Athletes should be aware of these possibilities, however rare they may be. They should recognize that suggestions for drug use by a coach or staff person are never justified and are a coaching abuse. The athlete should never put a physician in a position to compromise good medical care and judgment for the sake of an individual competition.

PEER PRESSURE

Pressure from peers is a primary incentive for using drugs. Because of trust in friends, the desire to be accepted, or a fear of being mocked or teased by or isolated from friends,

Why Athletes Do Drugs

refusing an invitation by peers to try drugs is extremely difficult.

Peer pressure is no less prevalent among athletes. In fact athletes, especially those involved in team sports, are very often close to their teammates. As one of the high school football players said of his own multiple drug use:

> It became more important for me to go out and get stoned with my buddies than to go to a picnic with my family.[1]

It is natural and easy to trust a teammate who tells you about the benefits of a drug. It is very uncomfortable and difficult to doubt, disagree, or contradict that friend. At times it is not easy to become accepted as part of the team. While acceptance and friendship should be based on motivation, contribution, and personality/behavior, if drugs are made part of the acceptance rite, refusing them can be very hard.

Finally, there may be pressure from a peer to "do it for the team." In an important competition, using anything that might help the team by enhancing one's performance may seem very inviting, loyal, and reasonable. Whether drug use can really help performance (or the team) is an issue that is open to question and will be discussed later. Athletes should be aware when they are being asked to compromise their own beliefs and principles, and, probably, their health. This is an unfair request and they should refuse.

MEDIA PRESSURE

The media (newspapers, television, radio, magazines), and sports have had a long relationship, one that has been good for sports and for athletes. They have reported results and developments in the field. They have made sports accessible to millions of people who otherwise could not enjoy them. In all likelihood, the media have been a major contributor to the growth and popularity of sports, and they have enabled athletes to become heroes. Television coverage, in particular, has allowed athletes to share in the rich rewards of sports. But the media can be a factor in drug abuse in sports.

For all these positive effects on sports, the media can contribute to the tremendous pressure on athletes. The simple fact is that publicity increases expectations. The manner of reporting is crucial as well. The media can sometimes "hype" or increase the importance of a competition beyond its actual significance.

A recent Olympics provided a good example of media pressure. The United States ice hockey team was rumored capable of beating the Russian team for the first time ever. The media hammered away at the potential victory so much that it was never absent from the public eye. The media made the fans believe that such a "miracle" was about to occur.

Just imagine the pressure. And after having built up such great expectations, the media was not very supportive of the team after it lost a game. After this loss the media immediately questioned the team's ability, even though that ability had been touted primarily by the media, not by the team. Despite the fact that team members were barely more than 18 years old, interviewers frequently asked them what it would feel like to disappoint the entire country! As if the pressure of being in the Olympics was not enough, the media turned victory into a national cause. Fortunately, the team came through. It seems unlikely, however, that the media pressure helped team members' confidence.

The media can focus on a player and keep him under the microscope of public scrutiny, or they can drop him from public recognition at a moment's notice. But the media have a more general effect on substance use as well. For example, commercials on television, the purpose of which is to change behavior and encourage people to buy or use the product being highlighted, often directly or indirectly portray substance abuse in a favorable light. In advertisements for alcohol, sports often play a large role. For example, one observer noted that one out of every 4.2 commercials during televised sport events advertised beer. In addition, professional athletes appeared in 90 percent of the ads for a low-calorie beer. Other substances, such as chewing tobacco, appear in similar ads. This situation seems to imply sports figures' endorsement, if not encouragement, of the use of such substances.

Another influence is that of star athletes who admit to using drugs. The media carry such statements and interviews and communicate them to millions of people and athletes alike. The media also carry stories of drug problems among athletes and teams. Although it is certainly the media's job to provide such information, depending on the attitude of the player interviewed and the slant of the story being reported, an impression might be left that drug abuse is a curiosity or a thrilling experience. Not all media sources have the integrity and professionalism to present the story objectively instead of in a manner designed to boost sales.

A final related influence is the proliferation of incomplete information or pseudoscientific articles about athlete performance enhancement. Athletes generally look for ways to improve their performance. Many people are willing to provide this information—usually at a cost—but not all of them are qualified to do so. Even quality media sources sometimes jump on a story so quickly that some facts may be misconstrued or the data may be incomplete. This may present a misleading view of the effectiveness and drawbacks of a particular procedure or substance. Of more concern is the almost unlimited array of information peddled to athletes and coaches about performance enhancement. While some of this information is very good, some may have little scientific basis. Myths, half-truths, and errors can be perpetuated for a long time.

It is up to the athlete to be sure that any training regimen, nutrition program, or other approach is based on good scientific data. With any technique, but especially with drug information, it is important to ask whether the information is reliable. How do you as an athlete judge reliability?

It is impossible to tell you how to evaluate scientific research here. But there are some basic questions you should ask before you accept information about drug effects as true. These are found in Table 6-2.

RECREATION AND EXPERIMENTATION
The so-called recreational use of drugs is a common introduction to excessive use and abuse. Drugs are used to elicit pleasurable feelings, to relax, and because they may make the user have feelings of efficiency and mastery. Athletes are not removed from the desire to "feel good" and experience these other altered mood states.

Ask the source of the information about drug effects:
   1 Is the information the result of scientific study or
      is it someone's opinion?

If it is an opinion:
   1 Does the person have any expertise about drugs?
   2 Are there any studies or other research to back up
      this opinion?

If it is a study:
   1 Is there more than one study that comes up with
      the same results?
   2 Where was the study done and by whom?
   3 How many athletes/people were studied?
   4 Are there any studies that resulted in different
      conclusions?
   5 What are the limitations of the study?

How to Judge the Accuracy of Information About Drug Effects

Table 6-2

Drugs are often first tried as an experiment—just to "see what it's all about." Sometimes, they are taken on a dare initially as part of a "game of chicken." Athletes may be particularly susceptible to these reasons for trying drugs.

Most athletes are in good, if not superb, physical shape. They may feel, therefore, that they are safe from whatever harm the drugs may cause. One time can't hurt, they think. They may feel invulnerable, which makes drug use *seem* harmless.

Athletes are also by definition competitors. Passing up a challenge, especially a dare, may be very difficult, even if it involves drug use. A false sense of security and a competitive nature can lead an athlete to experiment.

PERSONAL PROBLEMS

For a long time it was believed that athletes were more psychologically stable than nonathletes. While athletes may have some psychological strengths, which allow them to train hard and effectively, it is not clear that they are psychologically superior. Stress and personal and psychological problems can effect an athlete as much as anyone else. And just as the nonathlete population can turn to drugs to escape from personal problems, so can the athlete.

Stress and psychological problems can certainly be related to sports performance. An injury or a slump can be so devastating that the athlete searches for a magic cure. Another major stress for an athlete is the realization that hopes or goals are out of reach—there may be others who are just better. Unfortunately, very few athletes can become, by definition, number one, so second best (if that good) is a fate most will have to accept. Even worse may be the fear of being cut or eliminated when elite levels of competition are reached. A related situation for the experienced athlete is the end of a sports career whether through retirement, replacement, or injury.

In all of these situations the pressure to succeed remains, however. The essence of this has been captured by the athletic director of the University of North Dakota at Grand Forks, who is quoted as saying:

> ". . . .The day comes when the coach has to tell him. Meanwhile, of course, the kid is under enormous pressure to succeed, from his pals, his girlfriend, from everybody—nobody can face failure in our society. . . ."[2]

Drugs may be sought to ease the pain of such disappointments.

An athlete is a person, too. He has a personal life in addition to his athletic endeavors. There may be stresses, pressures, disappointments, conflicts, family worries, personal, school, or work problems. The survey of high school coaches in Pennsylvania (see Chapter 5) found that a significant number of athletes had personal problems apart from performance pressures.

Balancing an athletic career and its stringent demands with other aspects of life can be difficult indeed. Because athletes are expected to be strong, they may find it particularly difficult to admit when they are having problems. They may be afraid of being seen as weak or crazy, being laughed at or ridiculed. So, rather than seek help, they may try other less effective and more dangerous ways of coping.

The recent tragic case of a talented middle-distance college runner demonstrates the problem of stress among athletes. A female college junior had recently set a U.S. record in middle-distance competition. In 1986, apparently because of the pressure of her athletic, academic, and personal responsibilities and expectations, she suddenly bolted from the race in which she was competing at the NCAA Championships. She continued running out of the stadium to the nearest bridge and jumped off. Although her suicide attempt failed, she is now paralyzed in the lower half of her body.

Other athletes may have turned to drug use to cope. No athlete should ever reach the point where suicide or drug use is seen as the only way to handle personal problems. Help is available and should be sought long before such drastic actions are even considered.

ENABLERS

Although the decision is a personal one, drug use and abuse rarely begins as a solitary activity. The first impetus to try drugs may come from other people. Education about how to use drugs may come from others. The actual drugs may come from others.

After drug use and abuse has begun, others may still be needed to maintain the habit. People who make it possible for someone to continue to use drugs are sometimes called enablers.

Athletes have enablers too. Two types will be discussed here—the rescuer and the supplier. The rescuer protects the athlete from the consequences of drug use. Rescuers cover up for the athlete, make excuses for him, even lie for him. Rescuers may stay with the athlete when he is too strung out to function himself. Finally, rescuers may help to support the athlete's denial of a drug problem by agreeing that it really isn't abuse, that the athlete can handle it, that he can kick it tomorrow, that it will be okay, etc. Unfortunately, enablers are often the people closest to the athlete—a best friend, a family member, a girl or boyfriend. They are often people who *think* they are helping the athlete by shielding him from dealing realistically with the problem.

Another obvious enabler is the supplier, a connection for the drugs. It may simply be a fan or friend who gives drugs to the athlete. By supplying the athlete, these enablers may feel close to the athlete, boast of knowing him, and feel part of the glory. Unfortunately, they are destroying the athlete. Determining who really cares about you as a person and an athlete is an important skill for you to learn and one that will be discussed later.

Chapter Seven

The Case Against Drugs in Sports:
SOME THINGS TO CONSIDER

http://web3

The Case Against Drugs in Sports:

SOME THINGS TO CONSIDER   With all the reasons for athletes to use drugs, you may wonder why all athletes don't use them. They don't because there are a number of reasons why drugs and sport don't mix (see Table 7-1).

DRUG ABUSE IS HAZARDOUS TO YOUR HEALTH.
Perhaps the primary reason for an athlete not to use drugs without medical supervision is the risk they pose to the athlete's health. Physical condition is the most important prerequisite for athletic success, so that the health danger posed by drugs should be enough to make athletes avoid them.

Use of illicit drugs does threaten an athlete's health. Drug use is a threat in both the short term (acute use) and the long term (chronic use). It is a threat both physically and psychologically. Health dangers from either a single dose or from prolonged use are discussed in detail in chapter 8. For now suffice it to say that health risks range from decreased physical performance, to damage to the body's organs, to loss of sexual interest, to convulsions, to hallucinations, to death. Addiction is always a distinct possibility. A shortened athletic career, decreased motivation, and loss of concentration are common.

Consider the tragedy of Maryland basketball star, Len Bias. A June 30, 1986, article in *Sports Illustrated* said:

1 Drug abuse is hazardous to your health

2 Anticipated drug effects are not proven

3 Drug effects are variable and inconsistent

4 Drug use in sports cancels itself out

5 Drug use in sports is ethically wrong

6 Drug use demeans sports

7 Drug use demeans the athlete as an athlete

8 Drug use demeans the athlete as a person

9 Drug use in sports exposes athletes to danger from others

10 Drug use is illegal

The Case Against Using Drugs in Sport

Table 7-1

There wasn't a happier young athlete in America than Len Bias on the afternoon of June 17th. The NBA draft in New York City's Felt Forum was only 10 minutes old when the NBA Commissioner David Stern called Bias's name. As expected, the University of Maryland All American, a prototype NBA small forward who played with both power and finesse, had been summoned by the World Champion Boston Celtics as the second pick in the draft.

As Bias walked to the podium, someone handed him a green Celtics cap. He put it on and smiled shyly. For months Bias had been confiding to those close to him his dream of playing for the Celtics, and during a visit to Boston Garden for Game 1 of the NBA finals on May 26 he seemed almost transfixed as he sat at courtside. Well-muscled and 6'8", Bias had the talent and even the temperament—he was unfailingly irritating to opponents—to become the perfect Celtic. "Lenny had fallen in love with the idea of being a Celtic," Boston coach K.C. Jones would say later . . .

About 40 hours later, Bias, 22, was dead of cardiorespiratory arrest brought on by the use of cocaine, according to information related by the state medical examiner to SI on Monday. The heart of the man described by former Duke forward Mark Alarie as 'the best athlete I've ever seen, and that includes Michael Jordan,' had failed him. So, evidently, had Bias's good judgment, for he had been known as someone who avoided drugs . . .

ANTICIPATED DRUG EFFECTS ARE NOT PROVEN.
Much of what circulates in the sports community about the effects of drugs on performance is hearsay, myth, and incom-

plete, if not totally wrong. Scientific studies have shown that many of the touted effects of drugs on performance do not actually occur. Other studies show that such effects occur, not because of the drug, but because athletes *believed* they would occur and performed as if they had. For many other drugs, the scientific data on performance effects simply are not clear or do not exist yet.

Therefore, athletes cannot be sure that a drug will provide the supposed effect. They cannot know more than scientific data, which are often nonexistent. Most athletes do not bother to read the scientific data; instead they accept hearsay. In fact, one study found that most athletes never even bother to find out about the drug regulations that pertain to their sport.

It is not clear that a drug will enhance one's performance, so it is a risky bet in view of the clear health dangers.

DRUG EFFECTS ARE VARIABLE AND INCONSISTENT.

Even if a drug has been shown to have an effect on performance, the individual athlete has no guarantee that that is how he will react to the drug. Many factors influence how a drug affects performance. These include: one's unique physiology, the quantity and purity of the drug used, the time of day it is used, the presence of food in the stomach, level of fatigue, the degree of physical conditioning, use of other medications, general state of health, psychological state and expectation that the drug will work. This variability from individual to individual makes the use of drugs in sport a real long shot.

DRUG USE IN SPORTS CANCELS ITSELF OUT.

Let us assume for a moment that the performance-enhancing effects of drugs were absolute and consistent, and that drug use was safe and legal. What would happen? Most athletes would use drugs. What would this mean? Two athletes in competition would both use a drug before an event and achieve the same performance-enhancing results. What would be the deciding factor in victory? If drug effects were exactly predictable and the same, it would still be the training, talent, motivation, desire, and work of the individual athlete. The use of the drug by each athlete would cancel out use by the other.

There would be no advantage, the effect would be zero.

The idea has been captured in this rhyme about the use of the anabolic steroid Dianabol:

> Dianabol, Dianabol
> It's the gateway to fame.
> With Dianabol you'll win them all
> Unless the others are using the same.[1]

Thus, even though drug effects are *not* absolute, consistent, or safe, this cancellation factor still remains if two competitors use a drug. Therefore, although no probable advantage will be gained, much will be risked.

DRUG USE IN SPORTS IS ETHICALLY WRONG.

Sports are based on certain rules and assumptions. The rules of the game allow sports to exist by insuring fair competition so that the best can be judged as the best. These assumptions make sports a worthwhile endeavor. Drug use contradicts the rules and assumptions of sports and, therefore, is ethically wrong. The rules of sports do not allow drug use. The assumptions of sports do not condone it.

The ethical problem of drug use in sport has been described this way:

> If I said I could put the shot 90 feet with the aid of a sling or 2 miles with a cannon, you would rightly tell me I have missed the point of sport.[2]

If your opponent entered a swim meet with a jet ski, or a bicycle race with a motorcycle, you would contest this as giving him an unfair advantage. Drugs are the same kind of artificial manipulation of sport performance. To put it another way:

> In our conception of excellence in sport, some things are permissible, like expert coaching or exercise machines, and some things are not, like springs in shoes or drug-aided performance.[3]

There is another ethical problem with drug use in sports. When it is known that an athlete uses drugs to compete, it plants the idea *in the minds of opponents* that he has an edge and that if the opponents want to equalize the competition, they must use drugs as well. (Notice it was said *in the minds of opponents* for, as discussed earlier, drug-induced advantages are not guaranteed.)

Thus, using drugs coerces other athletes into thinking about or actually using them as well, something they might not normally consider. It is ethically wrong to pressure someone into an act against his will that is, a danger to himself and illegal.

DRUG USE DEMEANS SPORTS.

Drug use is not condoned in our society. Although there are inconsistencies in attitudes toward drug use and abuse, most people see drug abuse in a negative light. Therefore, as drug use permeates sports, sports themselves will share that negative reputation. Sporting accomplishment will be questioned and fans will become skeptical. Already a number of sports writers have said cynically that medals in competitive sport should be given to the drug companies and not the athletes.

DRUG USE DEMEANS THE ATHLETE AS AN ATHLETE.

Athletes *are* sports. If the public comes to see sports in a negative light because of drug use, that negative attitude will be applied to the athlete as well. The fans' respect for the athlete's accomplishments and victories is greatly reduced.

How will you defend yourself when it is said that drug use and not you, the athlete, are responsible for the performance? Perhaps, even worse, how will you be sure yourself that it was indeed you and not the drug that was responsible for your performance? Will you really feel entitled to your victory and your medal? A chemically derived victory is an artificial hollow victory. Is it any victory at all? Perhaps this is why most athletes are not against drug testing and measures and sanctions to help keep drugs out of sports.

DRUG USE DEMEANS THE ATHLETE AS A PERSON.

It must be remembered that athletes have a life apart from sports. You are a person as well as being an athlete. Drug use can affect both of these spheres. A negative reputation from athletic life can follow an athlete into his private life. The problems and dangers of drug use in sports contaminate private life as well. This is not a matter of a game or a performance; this is the rest of your life. Long after athletic glories have faded, fans remember drug use and drug reputations.

Joseph Pursch, medical director of Comprehensive Care Corporation, a California drug and alcohol care center, summarizes the point this way:

> "The problem with all drugs is that they make you feel like more than you are. If you need cocaine to make you feel like a bright basketball star, you are a dummy. If you need 'speed' to make you feel like a great football player, you ought to get out of the game."[4]

DRUG USE IN SPORTS EXPOSES ATHLETES TO DANGER FROM OTHERS.

In addition to risks to physical health posed by using drugs in sports, there are social dangers as well. Because drugs are illegal, they must be procured in precarious circumstances. This often brings the athlete into contact with undesirable individuals and criminals, and places him in dangerous situations. The need for money to pay for drugs also can lead to dangerous and illegal behavior.

Athletes are desirable targets for drug pushers because of the associated glories, contacts, and financial guarantees. Athletes have a lot to lose, once hooked, and pushers know this. Perhaps the worst squeeze of all is the athlete who is told to throw a game in order to obtain needed drugs or to forgive money that is owed.

DRUG USE IS ILLEGAL.

If the risks to health and physical danger are not enough, this reason should be first and sufficient to dissuade an athlete from drug use. Drug use is *ILLEGAL.* It is against the rules governing sports, and it is against the governing rules of society. There are sanctions by sports against drug use among athletes that can hurt a career. There are also sanctions against drug use by society that can ruin your life.

For example, federal law says that the first-time conviction for possession of cocaine is punishable by imprisonment for up to one year, a fine of $5,000, or both. A first offense for trafficking in cocaine is imprisonment up to 15 years, a fine up to $125,000, or both. If the infraction occurs within 1,000 feet of a school, the maximum penalties can be doubled.

There is another important implication of the illegality of drugs besides that of punishment: the purity of drugs bought illegally cannot be assured. In fact, most street drugs are not pure; they have been adulterated. Street cocaine is generally only 12 percent to 75 percent pure and amphetamines are reported now to be only 12 percent to 15 percent pure.

If you are lucky, street drugs are diluted with only harmless substances like sugar, which stretch the quantity of the drug and make more of a profit for the dealer. Unfortunately, a variety of other stimulants or drugs are mixed with little regard to what effect they will have on the user. That's when the danger to the athlete's health becomes more likely.

Chapter Eight

Drugs: The Good and the Bad
AN ATHLETE'S RESOURCE SECTION

Drugs: The Good and the Bad

AN ATHLETE'S RESOURCE SECTION

In this chapter, special attention is given to the specific drugs themselves. Before an athlete decides to take a drug, he should find out the answers to the questions listed in Table 8-1.

It is impossible to catalogue every abused drug and its effects here. Instead, those categories of drugs most likely to be used by athletes are included. Before the categories are presented, it is useful to give some general definitions to common terms that are used when discussing drug use and abuse.

1 DRUG ADDICTION: a state resulting from the continued use of a drug with the following characteristics: (a) an overpowering need to continue using the drug and obtain it whatever the means or cost; (b) a tendency to use increasing doses of the drug; (c) occurrence of symptoms when use of the drug is discontinued; (d) such withdrawal symptoms stop if the drug is taken again; (e) a psychological craving or need for the drug; and (f) detrimental effects to the individual and society.

2 DRUG ABUSE: the persistent and usually excessive use of a drug leading to the potential for addiction, physical or psychological harm, and/or social problems, and where the use is different from the typical social pattern of society.

3 ABSTINENCE OR WITHDRAWAL SYNDROME: a series of unpleasant symptoms that occur when a drug

1 Definition, description of the drug

2 What is the history of the drug?

3 What are the accepted medical uses of the drug?

4 What are the physical, psychological, and behavioral effects of the drug?

5 What are the side effects of the drug?

6 What are the toxic effects of the drug?

7 What is the tolerance potential of the drug?

8 What is the addiction potential of the drug?

9 How does the drug affect sports performance?

10 What is the legal status of the drug?

What Athletes Should Know Before Even Considering Use of a Drug for Sport

Table 8-1

that has been used for some time is discontinued (usually suddenly); generally the effects are relieved by using the drug again.

4 DOPING: the administration to or use by a competing athlete of any substance foreign to the body or of any physiological substance taken in abnormal quantity or taken by an abnormal route of entry into the body, with the sole intention of increasing in an artificial manner performance in competition.

5 DRUG CROSS-TOLERANCE: a situation where the use of one drug creates tolerance to other drugs of a similar nature or class (see definition of drug tolerance, below).

6 DRUG DEPENDENCE: a general term for a state of psychological or physical dependence (need) or both, arising in an individual after using a drug over a period of time or on a continuous basis.

7 DRUG POTENTIATION: a situation where using one drug increases or exaggerates the effects of another drug.

8 DRUG SCHEDULE: categorization of drugs by the federal government on the basis of use, abuse, and control. The schedules are as follows:

Schedule I—drugs that have a high potential for abuse and have no current medical use in the u.s.

Schedule II—drugs that have a high abuse potential that may lead to a severe dependence. They have a current accepted therapeutic use, but a special written prescription must be used.

Schedule III—drugs that have a lower abuse potential than Schedule I or II drugs. Abuse of these drugs can lead to moderate or physical dependence or high levels of psychological dependence. A prescription is needed.

Schedule IV—drugs with low abuse potential, and whose abuse leads to limited physical or psychological dependence. A prescription is needed.

Schedule V—drugs with a lower abuse potential than Schedule IV and only limited psychological or physical dependence. No prescription is needed for many of these drugs but the buyer's name is entered in a log book.

9 DRUG TOLERANCE: the adaptation of the body to the effects of a drug so that higher and higher amounts or doses of the drug are required to achieve the same effects.

10 DRUG TOXICITY: the amount and effects from a single dose or chronic use of a drug that are high enough to produce uncomfortable or life-endangering symptoms.

11 OVER-THE-COUNTER DRUGS: any of the variety of drugs or preparations that can be obtained without a physician's prescription at a pharmacy, retail store, etc.

12 PLACEBO EFFECT: expected effects that occur when a drug (or inert substance) is used, which are not the result of the drug itself (or the inert substance), but rather the person's belief and expectation that the effects will occur.

13 PRESCRIPTION DRUGS: drugs which by law (federal, state, or both) can be obtained only with a physician's written prescription.

14 PSYCHOLOGICAL DEPENDENCE: the state where discontinued use of a drug or continuous use of a drug creates an overwhelming desire, need, and craving for more of the drug.

15 SIDE EFFECTS: undesirable and unwanted results that can occur in susceptible people when using a drug, even in the manner intended.

The remainder of this chapter lists the categories of drugs deemed of special interest to athletes; their use and history; their symptoms and effects on the body; their trade and generic name. It also describes the United States Olympic Committee/International Olympic Committee (USOC/IOC) and National Collegiate Athlete Association (NCAA) stands on their use (see Table 8-21 for a summary.)[1]

ALCOHOL

Alcohol use (and abuse) in most societies is so common that people often forget that alcohol is a drug. Alcohol comes in many different forms, including beers, table wines, cocktail or dessert wines, liqueurs or cordials, and distilled spirits. The history of alcohol is probably as long as history itself. Its prominent role is characterized by the fact that in the Middle Ages it was called "elixir of life," and the term whiskey comes from the Gaelic term for "water of life."

Alcohol has been used for a variety of medical purposes: as an antiseptic, as a solvent for other substances, for stimulation of appetite in certain elderly or debilitated patients, and in control of pain.

Alcohol has significant physical effects. It lowers body temperature, but it can also lead to temperature regulation problems, such as a fever in a hotter than normal environment. Alcohol does not warm the body on a cold day, as is often believed. It dilates the peripheral blood vessels, which gives an initial feeling of warmth. However, dilation of the blood vessels actually leads to more rapid heat loss and a decrease in body temperature.

Alcohol's direct effect on the heart tends to be minimal. There appears to be little evidence to support alcohol as a vasodilator (which increases blood flow) to the coronary arteries. Alcohol is an irritant to the stomach and prolonged intoxication can shut down the entire gastrointestinal tract. Alcohol acts as a diuretic. Effects on the liver tend to be detrimental and are discussed below.

It is the psychological and behavioral effects of alcohol that are best known and most dramatic. Although alcohol appears to be a stimulant because of the behavior it unleashes, it is actually a depressant. The increase in volatile behavior occurs because of alcohol's depressant effect on the "control" portions of the brain.

Alcohol affects self-restraint first. The user feels a false sense of confidence. Discrimination and judgment become impaired as do memory, concentration, and insight. Mood swings and emotional outbursts can occur. Such effects are more prevalent when alcohol levels are rising, rather than falling.

Dying to Win

The negative effects of chronic alcohol use and abuse range from mild to severe physical changes. An increase in caloric intake, and a resulting weight gain are common, especially with beer. However, alcohol is not a good source of nutrition and, in fact, chronic use can lead to severe nutritional deficiencies.

Peripheral nerve damage (peripheral polyneuropathies) occurs. Cirrhosis of the liver can result, as can cardiac and skeletal muscle damage. Alcohol has significant detrimental effects during pregnancy, including an increased number of stillbirths and spontaneous abortions. Infants whose mothers have consumed excessive amounts of alcohol during gestation often have lowered birth weight and developmental problems, known as fetal alcohol syndrome.

Alcoholism is related to many other detrimental effects, such as accidents, lost productivity, broken homes, and interrupted lives.

Most of the effects seen with alcohol, such as the behavior changes, represent toxic levels of alcohol in the blood and body. The effects are dose-related. The lowest levels of concentration (blood alcohol levels of .03 percent to .05 percent) produce lowered alertness. However, it is at this level that the good feeling occurs and people become outgoing and gregarious. As the level rises, there are large consistent increases in reaction time, and people become less cautious. At a blood alcohol level of .20 percent, there is a marked decrease in sensory and motor abilities; the person is decidedly intoxicated and may feel dizzy and exhibit disturbing behavior. At slightly higher levels, there is severe motor disturbance, staggering, a feeling of being smashed; behavior can be repugnant and the person disheveled-looking. At blood alcohol levels of .30 percent to .35 percent the person moves from semi-stupor to being dead drunk. Surgical anesthesia levels are reached, which is near the lower lethal level, about .40 percent blood alcohol level. Death is likely when the blood alcohol level reaches .60 percent. Life-threatening events occur more readily and often by accident when alcohol is mixed with the use of other pills such as depressants.

Some tolerance to alcohol occurs over time, although there is no tolerance to the lethal level. The major concern with alcohol use is addiction. Withdrawal from chronic alcohol use has been described as consisting of three states or stages.

A few hours after the last drink there is tremulousness, which may be mild or so severe that the person cannot lift or hold objects. There is nausea, weakness, anxiety, sweating, cramps, and vomiting. People start to see things. This occurs, at first, only when the eyes are closed; then it happens even when the eyes are open.

Withdrawal progresses to the second stage—hallucinations, which may be accompanied by seizures.

Delirium tremens (DTS) is the final stage. In the DTS, people cannot sleep; they are agitated, disoriented, confused, and terrified by auditory, visual, and/or tactile hallucinations. Fever, profound perspiration, and tachycardia (quickened heartrate) occur. The DTS, which are also known as "the horrors" can last for three to four days. Death is not infrequent during this stage for a variety of reasons, including hypothermia, vascular problems, and self-inflicted injury.

Alcohol affects athletic performance negatively. Some people believe that small quantities of alcohol can aid muscle endurance slightly, but this has been challenged and critiqued. Some think that alcohol is a good source of energy, which is also false. The best view of alcohol in terms of athletic performance is that it is a deconditioner. Its use leaves the central nervous system irritable and it has toxic muscle effects. It increases reaction time, impairs skills, and endangers health. Alcohol taken the night before competition decreases performance the next day. A summary of the effects of alcohol use in sports has been provided recently by a position statement from the American College of Sports Medicine (a national association of sports scientists). The College concluded in 1982, after looking at the scientific evidence, that:

1 The acute ingestion of alcohol can exert a deleterious effect upon a wide variety of psychomotor skills, such as reaction time, and eye coordination, accuracy, balance, and complex coordination.

2 Acute ingestion of alcohol will not substantially influence the metabolic or physiological functions essential to physical performance, such as energy metabolism,

maximal oxygen consumption (VO_2 max), heart rate, stroke volume, cardiac output, muscle blood flow, arterio-venous oxygen difference, or respiratory dynamics. Alcohol consumption may impair body temperature regulation during prolonged exercise in a cold environment.

3 Acute alcohol ingestion will not improve and may decrease strength, power, local muscular endurance, speed and cardiovascular endurance.

4 Alcohol is the most abused drug in the United States and is a major contributing factor to accidents and their consequences. Also, it has been documented widely that prolonged excessive alcohol consumption can elicit pathological changes in the liver, heart, brain, and muscle, which can lead to disability and death.

5 Serious and continuing effort should be made to educate athletes, coaches, health and physical educators, physicians, trainers, sports media, and the general public regarding the effects of acute alcohol ingestion upon human physical performance and on the potential acute and chronic problems of excessive alcohol consumption.

Alcohol is, of course, illegal for use by minors and is governed by the laws of various states. It is not on the United States Olympic Committee's or the International Olympic Committee's (USOC/IOC) banned drug list, but can be and is tested for at some international competitions. It is on the NCAA's doping list for specific sports.

Drugs: The Good and the Bad

AMPHETAMINES

The term amphetamines refers to a group of chemically-related drugs that have a stimulant effect on the brain and body. They share similarities to sympathomimetic drugs discussed in a later section. The more common amphetamines are benzedrine (amphetamine), dexedrine (dextroamphetamine), methedrine (methamphetamine), and the related drug, Ritalin (methylphenidate). A more complete listing is presented in Table 8-2. The amphetamines go by many different street names: bennies, benz, black beauties, chicken patter, crank, crystal, dex, dexies, eye-openers, goof balls, greenies, jolly beans, meth, oranges, pep pills, pills, sparklers, uppers, ups, and speed.

Table 8-2
Representative Amphetamine-Like Drugs

Generic Name	Trade Name
amphetamine	Benzedrine
dextroamphetamine	Dexedrine
dextroamphetamine + amobarbital	Dexamyl
dextroamphetamine + amphetamine	Diphetamine
methamphetamine	Methadrine Desoxyn
methylphenidate	Ritalin
phenmetrazine	Preludin

Amphetamines are generally synthetic drugs, created in a laboratory. Amphetamines were first synthesized in 1887 by a German scientist. The drugs have had a long history of medical uses, many of which are no longer continued or appropriate.

Amphetamines were "rediscovered" in the 1930s, when it was found that the drugs could raise blood pressure. Amphetamines were also marketed in a nasal inhaler to be used to shrink the mucous membranes of the nose for congestion due to colds, hay fever, and asthma. They were also used in the past for the treatment of schizophrenia; addiction to morphine, codeine, nicotine, caffeine; for sea sickness; for heart block, etc. Because they were thought to be harmless and not addicting initially, they were given freely to soldiers during World War II as pep pills. Amphetamine abuse has also been popularized by truck drivers, students, and housewives.

The current medical uses of amphetamines are now greatly reduced and limited to only a few situations. Narcolepsy, a syndrome of severe attacks of sleepiness and lost muscle tone occurring throughout the day, is one area of use on a short-term basis. Ritalin is used to help children who are hyperactive or who have attention deficit disorders. There are a few limited circumstances where amphetamines may be used for depression, but they generally only increase motor behavior and do not lift the mood of the depressed person. There are more efficient medications for this purpose. Finally, there is the controversial short-term use of amphetamines to aid weight loss, since amphetamines reduce appetite. How effective, safe, and abuse-free the amphetamines are for the purpose of weight loss is open to much questioning, however.

The physical effects of amphetamines include a rise in blood pressure and, in higher doses, a rise in the rate and force of cardiac contractions. They also cause dilated pupils, dry mouth, increased breathing rate, and increased use of the body's stored energy. Weight loss is common. Also common is the wearing of sunglasses due to light sensitivity from dilated pupils.

Behaviorally, amphetamines increase physical activity and produce restlessness. Excessive talking, especially at an increased rate and on many different topics, often occurs. Psychologically, amphetamines make a person feel good about his abilities and increase self-esteem and self-confidence. Increased alertness and euphoria from the drug makes individuals *feel* that they can perform better; however, this is generally not the case. Amphetamines improve performance of simple repetitive tasks, such as sorting and stapling pages together, because there is some relief from fatigue. The warding off of fatigue, however, is short-lived and a person may feel more

Drugs: The Good and the Bad

alert, but actually have impaired judgment and slower reaction time.

The use and misuse of amphetamines can create a variety of problems. The effect of a single excessive dose can include headaches, excessive sweating, dry mouth, large pupils, a rapid but weak heartbeat, tremors of the fingers and hands, rapid breathing, nausea, dizziness, increased blood pressure, and irregular heartbeats. Death can also occur. An increase in sexual desire is reported at low doses, but there is a decrease in sexual performance at higher doses.

More chronic use can cause damage to the blood vessels. By obscuring fatigue and pain levels, amphetamines can allow the athlete to "run the red light" and continue to perform in a manner that may lead to more severe and permanent injuries.

Chronic use can also lead to amphetamine psychosis, a paranoid state where the person feels everyone is out to get him. Hallucinations of both a visual and auditory nature can occur. There are also tactile hallucinations, such as feeling small animals brushing against the skin or crystals under the skin. People may use knives or razor blades to cut away the perceived irritation, creating much damage, or may constantly pick and scratch.

Tolerance develops to the feelings of euphoria and well-being, so much that amphetamine abusers may increase their initial dose 50 to 100 times to try to get the effect again. Cardiac tolerance seems to develop because the normal heart could not survive the high doses that some abusers use.

Amphetamine addiction and withdrawal do occur. The withdrawal syndrome can range from mild discomfort to an overwhelming need for the drug. In the initial phase of withdrawal, an individual can sleep continuously for up to three days. Abnormalities in brain wave tests are seen. There may be increased appetite. There may be a state of depression lasting up to two weeks. In withdrawal, individuals can also experience irritability, apathy, anxiety, extreme fear, and obsessions. The symptoms are not relieved by taking more amphetamines. The additional and toxic hazard of chronic use is the abuse of alcohol and other depressants to counter the stimulating effects of amphetamines, leading to problems and/or withdrawal from both.

Amphetamine use in sports was once extremely widespread; they were commonly used by professional football teams in the 1960s and 1970s. Use was so common that it was called "the Sunday Syndrome." Amphetamines were used to help athletes ignore pain from injuries, overcome sleepiness caused by other pain-killing medications, and get "up" for the game. Greater control of amphetamines, more information on their toxic effects, as well as lawsuits against teams from players who were hooked on the drugs have led to a marked decrease in the open use of amphetamines.

It should be noted that the toxic effects of an acute dose of amphetamine can occur at much lower levels if the drug is combined with strenuous athletic training. Heat exhaustion and heat stroke during athletic activity in hot weather are more likely on amphetamines. In the 1967 Tour de France, a bicyclist collapsed in a coma and died during a 6,000-foot climb in 90° heat. Autopsy showed significant amounts of methamphetamine in his system.

The beneficial effect of amphetamines in sports is questionable. While physical effects certainly are produced by the use of amphetamines, increased athletic performance doesn't necessarily follow. On the other hand, some research has shown a small percentage of improvement in sports performance. Other studies have questioned this, and it also has been suggested that improvement tends to be variable and may be reversed by repeated "use" or overdosage. Some athletes have miscued or misfired because of being too "hepped up" on amphetamines and not being able to control their behavior. Thus, while performance might be enhanced, it also must be remembered that it is usually the *perception* of ability that is increased, that the effects are variable, and that there are dangerous side effects from the drug use.

Amphetamines are a highly controlled substance (Schedule II) and illegal, except by prescription. They are banned by the USOC, IOC, and NCAA.

ANABOLIC STEROIDS

Anabolic steroids are among the most controversial drugs in sports today. They have been known alternately as "the breakfast of champions" and "fool's gold."

Anabolic steroids are related to and synthesized from the male hormone testosterone. First synthesized in the 1950s, these drugs were found to increase weight and bulk in debilitated individuals. Apparently an American physician who was also a weightlifter reasoned that these bulking effects might also occur in nondebilitated individuals. He reportedly experimented on himself by taking anabolic steroids, discussed his experience in a weightlifting magazine, and started the anabolic steroid craze that still continues.

Medically, anabolic steroids are used to treat muscle-wasting diseases, where weight gain is desirable. They have a role in the treatment of metastatic cancer, aplastic anemia, and chronic renal failure. Anabolic steroids are also used to increase muscle mass in cattle meant for slaughter.

Interest in anabolic steroids by athletes has been extensive. It has been said that by the mid-1970s, some athletes were trading steroids or "schedules of use" among themselves instead of T-shirts. It also has been reported that virtually 100 percent of power athletes (weightlifters and shot-putters) believe contests are won not only on ability, but with the help of steroids as well. A recent survey found that 45 percent of athletes obtained their steroids illegally.

Why do athletes use anabolic steroids? Generally, to increase weight and strength. Athletes may feel that they can train harder when on steroids, and they often do. High dose steroids and heavy resistance training can yield an increase in body weight and muscle size, as well as in appetite and dietary intake. And there can also be an increase in aggression.

While this may sound promising, the positive effects of anabolic steroids are far from clear for many reasons. First, it is not known whether the increase in static strength actually leads to improved athletic performance. In fact, the whole issue of the effects of anabolic steroids is unclear. For example, normal, healthy men who take anabolic steroids without training show no effect on muscle size or strength. Some of the weight gain has been attributed to retained body water, rather than performance-related bulk.

While some studies have attempted to show positive effects from anabolic steroid use, the conclusions of these studies have been called into question. For example, even the so-called success studies show that the gains made by athletes taking anabolic steroids are very minimal compared to those athletes who did not take anabolic steroids. In other studies, those athletes *not* taking anabolic steroids showed more of the expected results than athletes who did take them. Studies have not shown conclusively that anabolic steroids increase lean muscle bulk and strength any more than simple weight resistance training alone.

There are scientific problems with many of the anabolic steroid studies, too. Often, too few athletes are studied to reach conclusions that are generally applicable. Other times, errors in calculation were found in the reported conclusions. In still other studies, important factors that also might account for the increased bulk—other than the drug use (like diet)—were not considered or controlled. While athletes often take very high doses of steroids, some studies showed gains on very low

Table 8-3

Representative Anabolic Steroids

Generic Name	Trade Name
ethylestrenol	Maxibolin
methandriol	Anabol, Andriol
methandriol dipropionate	Methabolic
methandrostenolone	Dianabol
methyltestosterone	Oreton
nandrolone decanoate	Deca-Durabolin, Hybolin
nandrolone phenpropionate	Durabolin, Nandrolin
oxymetholone	Anadrol-50
stanozolol	Winstrol

Drugs: The Good and the Bad

doses of steroids. There seems to be little relationship between the amount of anabolic steroid taken and the results achieved.

While tolerance and addiction are probably not as important an issue for anabolic steroids as for some other drugs, the toxic and side effects from use certainly are. This is especially true because there is no yardstick for a safe dose. While the recommended therapeutic dose is 2.5 to 10 mg/day, athletes often use 100 to 400 mg/day. Such use has many troubling consequences.

Salt and water retention produced by the drugs can lead to hypertension. Problems with hepatitis and jaundice can occur. Normal steroid production by the adrenal glands may be altered, resulting in a variety of endocrine problems. Of particular concern are reported cases of liver cancer in athletes using anabolic steroids. There may be a premature closing of the epiphyses, or bone plates, which can lead to stunted or retarded growth. When athletes go off anabolic steroids, they often feel depressed.

In female athletes, the use of anabolic steroids leads to masculinization. Body hair increases, and the voice deepens. Clitoral enlargement and menstrual irregularities can occur. While not proven, there has been speculation that excessively rapid aging, which was reported to occur in some women champions, may have been related to steroid use.

Males who use anabolic steroids can expect special difficulties as well. Problems with worsening acne and cholesterol build-up are found. Males also experience reduced sperm production and atrophy of the testicles. Kidney dysfunction, premature baldness, and prostate problems can occur. Natural testosterone levels are decreased. Gynecomastia, or the enlargement of the breasts, can occur. In fact, enlargement of the nipples and surrounding tissues is so well-recognized as a side effect that the condition has been given the name "bitch tits" by some athletes.

While many of these effects are reversible in the short-term, there are very few data on the chronic effects (those stemming from long-term use). Perhaps one sports medicine physician summed it up best when he said:

> When a young man asks me if he should use anabolic steroids, I tell him to reach into his pocket and ask himself if he wants to tamper with what he's got down there.[2]

Legally anabolic steroids are prescription drugs. They are on the USOC/IOC's and NCAA's list of banned doping substances. The American College of Sports Medicine (ACSM) and the American Academy of Pediatrics also have condemned the use of anabolic steroids. The ACSM recently revised its view of anabolic steroids in sports. While its position statement acknowledges that there may be an increase in body weight and strength under certain conditions in the presence of steroids, it further states that the health dangers are great and it clearly condemns steroid use in sports. The preamble to the ACSM position stand on anabolic steroids states:

> Based on a comprehensive literature survey and a careful analysis of the claims concerning the ergogenic effects and the adverse effects of anabolic-androgenic steroids, it is the position of the American College of Sports Medicine that:
>
> 1 Anabolic-androgenic steroids in the presence of an adequate diet can contribute to increases in body weight, often in the lean mass compartment.
>
> 2 The gains in muscular strength achieved through high-intensity exercise and proper diet can be increased by the use of anabolic-androgenic steroids in some individuals.
>
> 3 Anabolic-androgenic steroids do not increase aerobic power or capacity for muscular exercise.
>
> 4 Anabolic-androgenic steroids have been associated with adverse effects on the liver, cardiovascular system, reproductive system, and psychological status in therapeutic

trials and in limited research on athletes. Until further research is completed, the potential hazards of the use of the anabolic-androgenic steroids in athletes must include those found in therapeutic trials.

5 The use of anabolic-androgenic steroids by athletes is contrary to the rules and ethical principles of athletic competition as set forth by many of the sports governing bodies. The American College of Sports Medicine supports these ethical principles and deplores the use of anabolic-androgenic steroids by athletes.

This document is a revision of the 1977 position stand of the American College of Sports Medicine concerning anabolic-androgenic steroids. . . .

Perhaps the most telling is the fact that the *Physicians' Desk Reference,* a standard reference physicians use to check on drug effects, has carried the message: "Warning: anabolic steroids do not enhance athletic ability."

ANTIDEPRESSANT DRUGS

Antidepressant drugs were discovered in the late nineteenth century, but their mood-altering properties were not taken advantage of until the 1940s. Antidepressants are used in certain situations to treat people who are clinically depressed. Some of the drugs have a sedating effect, and certain specific drugs may be used in treating chronic pain. They may also be used in treating panic disorders, bulimia, and obsessive-compulsive states.

Antidepressant drugs generally elevate mood in a depressed individual. It is important to realize that antidepressants are not stimulants like amphetamines. The two drug groups often are confused, however. Just as stimulants do not have the antidepressant effect of mood elevation, antidepressants do not act as amphetamines to increase motor activity.

Table 8-4
Representative Antidepressant Drugs

Generic Names	Trade Names
Tricyclic Antidepressants:	
amitriptyline HCl	Amitril, Elavil
amoxapine	Asendin
desipramine HCl	Norpramin, Pertofrane
doxepin HCl	Adapin, Sinequan
imipramine HCl	Janimine, Tofranil
maprotiline HCl	Ludiomil
nortriptyline HCl	Aventyl, Pamelor
primipramine maleate	Surmontil
protriptyline HCl	Vivactil
Atypical Antidepressants:	
trazodone HCl	Desyrel
Monoamine Oxidase Inhibitors	
isocarboxazide	Marplan
pargyline HCl	Eutonyl
phenelzine sulfate	Nardil
tranylcypromine sulfate	Parnate

In fact, in nondepressed people, antidepressants cause one to feel sleepy, decrease blood pressure, and impart a feeling of lightheadedness. Gait can be unsteady, and the person can be clumsy and feel tired. There are also what are known as anticholinergic effects—dry mouth, blurred vision, constipation, and urinary retention. In general, the side effects of antidepressants in nondepressed people are unpleasant.

The side effects and toxic effects are basically those anticholinergic symptoms already described. Lowered blood pressure (hypotension) can also be a problem. There is also the possibility that antidepressants can cause disturbances in cardiac rhythm. At the higher and toxic levels, a sour metallic taste can occur, as can stomach distress, palpitations, and quickened heart rate (tachycardia). Weakness, fatigue, and excessive sweating are possible, and death from overdose can occur. It is also important to recognize that there are different types of antidepressants and particularly one subset, the MAO (monoamine oxidase) inhibitors, are especially prone to problematic side effects. In fact, individuals using MAO inhibitors have to avoid certain foods (including red wine and aged cheese) to prevent serious potential negative reactions.

Tolerance occurs to the anticholinergic side effects of the antidepressants. Addiction and withdrawal are generally not a problem. However, some people have reported malaise, chills, cold-like symptoms, or muscle aching when they stop using the drug.

Antidepressant drugs are prescription medications. They are banned in specific sports by the USOC and IOC. They are not banned by the NCAA.

ANTIPSYCHOTIC DRUGS/MAJOR TRANQUILIZERS

Antipsychotic drugs, or the major tranquilizers, were first developed in the 1950s. These drugs have very significant calming effects and are used mainly in treating psychosis, schizophrenia, and mania, as well as to control nausea and vomiting. The drugs are known as major tranquilizers because of their use in these more serious psychiatric disturbances, as compared to the benzodiazepines (sometimes known as minor tranquilizers), used in less severe (anxiety) situations.

The antipsychotic drugs decrease blood pressure, though generally there is relatively little direct cardiac effect. They also produce some skeletal muscle relaxation and decreased spontaneous motor activity; they can produce different kinds of movement disorders, and they have varying degrees of anticholinergic effects (dry mouth, urinary retention, etc.). In schizophrenic individuals, the major tranquilizers improve thought disorders and affect (emotions), reduce withdrawal, and help control hallucinations and hostility.

Negative effects of the major tranquilizers include the possibility of some cardiac rhythm disturbance, depressed mood, and difficulties with menstruation. At high levels, the antipsychotic drugs can produce symptoms of Parkinsonism (motor problems). There can also be aggressive behavior, impulsive actions, and psychotic symptoms, including delusions and hallucinations. Tremor, rigidity, and orthostatic hypotension (a drop in blood pressure on arising quickly) are possible. One very serious side effect of sustained use of high levels of antipsychotics is tardive dyskinesia—involuntary chewing and grimacing movements of the face and neck, which are often difficult, if not impossible, to treat or stop.

There is a modest tolerance to the sedating effect of these drugs. Addiction and withdrawal are generally not a problem with the major tranquilizers. However, symptoms of chronic use include lack of initiative, disinterest in the environment, and reduced emotional responses. The lethal dose is relatively high.

The major tranquilizers require a prescription for use, but are unscheduled drugs. They are banned in specific sports by the USOC and IOC but not by the NCAA.

Table 8-5
Representative Antipsychotic Drugs

Generic Name	Trade Name
chlorpromazine HCl	Thorazine
fluphenazine HCl	Prolixin, Permitil
haloperidol	Haldol
mesoridazine	Serentil
perphenazine	Trilafon
prochlorperazine	Compazine
promazine HCl	Sparine
thioridazine	Mellaril
trifluoperazine	Stelazine

BARBITURATES AND THE SEDATIVES AND HYPNOTICS

Sedatives are drugs that decrease activity, moderate excitement, and calm a person down. Hypnotics produce drowsiness and are used to promote sleep. These types of drugs have been the object of many fads and phases, beginning with chloral hydrate and paraldehyde, and bromides, the barbiturates, and—as will be discussed later—the tranquilizers or benzodiazepines. This section will focus on barbiturates.

Medically, barbiturates are used for sedation, sleep, and to control convulsions. Their use has been reduced markedly for two reasons. First, their effects are not very specific—they impair all activity, not just agitation. Second, their use for anxiety conditions has been reduced because more effective agents (the benzodiazepines) are now available.

In the street lingo of abuse, barbiturates are known as goof balls. Individual drugs have nicknames derived from their capsule colorings and properties. These include yellow jackets (pentobarbital), red devils (secobarbital), blue angels (Amytal), and rainbows (Tuinal).

The effect of the barbiturates at lower doses is to provide mild but generalized sedation. They depress gastrointestinal activity and respiration, and they affect the liver so that greater interaction with other drugs occurs. Toxic levels of barbiturates produce general sluggishness and slowed, slurred speech. There may be difficulty in thinking, poor comprehension and memory, and a narrow range of attention and faculty judgment. Emotional lability can occur, as can exaggeration of basic personality traits, irritability, quarrelsomeness, moroseness, untidiness, hostility, and paranoia. As doses increase, the brain can be depressed to anesthetic levels. Coma and death by respiratory/cardiac failure can occur.

Chronic misuse can lead to psychosis. Barbiturate "hangover" is also seen at higher doses, as is residual depression.

Tolerance develops to most actions of this class of drugs, particularly to mood and sedative effects. There is less tolerance to anticonvulsant and lethal effects. Coma, respiratory failure, shock, and death occur with excessive doses. For phenobarbital, this lethal range is six to ten grams, and for secobarbital and pentobarbital, the range is only two to three grams. Mixing barbiturates and alcohol significantly increases

Table 8-6
Representative Barbiturates and Related Compounds

Generic Name	Trade Name
amobarbital	Amytal
amobarbital + secobarbital	Tuinal
aprobarbital	Alurate
butabarbital	Butisol
pentobarbital	Nembutal
phenobarbital	Luminal
secobarbital	Seconal
talbutal	Lofusate

Related Compounds

Generic Name	Trade Name
chloral hydrate	Noctec
ethchlorvynol	Placidyl
glutethimide	Doriden
meprobamate	Miltown
paraldehyde	Paral

the depressive effects of both, and this unpredictable combination causes many deaths.

Addiction to barbiturates occurs. The symptoms of withdrawal are known as the "general depressant withdrawal syndrome." In its mild form, withdrawal consists of insomnia and anxiety. In its more severe form, there is tremor, weakness, and more pronounced anxiety and insomnia. In the severe form, tonic/clonic (grand mal or epilepsy-type convulsions) seizures can occur, as can delirium and visual hallucinations. Abdominal cramps, nausea, and vomiting are also part of the

Drugs: The Good and the Bad

picture. Cardiac collapse is possible. Babies born to addicted mothers go through withdrawal after birth.

In relation to sports performance, it is important to note that barbiturates impair judgment and fine motor skills. This is in addition to other relevant effects already noted above. Higher doses have been shown to impair driving and flying skills for as long as 10 to 22 hours.

Barbiturates are prescription drugs and their use is governed by various state laws. These drugs are banned in specific sports by the USOC and IOC. They are not banned by the NCAA.

BENZODIAZEPINES

The benzodiazepines are anti-anxiety and tranquilizing agents. They have replaced barbiturates as a preferred method of sedation and tranquilization. Benzodiazepines have a variety of medical uses in addition to their anti-anxiety role. They are used as anticonvulsants, pre-anesthetic medications and muscle relaxants, and for insomnia and alcohol withdrawal.

Their action is similar to that of barbiturates, in that they relieve tension and reduce anxiety. They have little effect on respiration unless there is a medical problem such as chronic

Table 8-7
Representative Benzodiazepines

Generic Name	Trade Name
alprazolam	Xanax
clorazepate dipotassium	Tranxene
chlordiazepoxide HCl	Librium
diazepam	Valium
flurazepam HCl	Dalmane
lorazepam	Ativan
oxazepam	Serax
temazepam	Restoril
triazolam	Halcion

obstructive pulmonary disease. They can have a calming effect on the gastrointestinal tract. Side effects include drowsiness, confusion, fatigue, weakness, unsteady gait, dizziness, headache, and tremor. Tolerance occurs to most effects of the benzodiazepines.

Toxic levels produce somnolence, confusion, coma, and diminished reflexes. Cardiac arrest has been reported, but is generally rare—unless drugs have been mixed with alcohol. Chronic use does lead to symptoms upon cessation. These can include insomnia, restlessness, dizziness, nausea, abdominal pain, paresthesias (tingling, numbness), headache, aggressiveness, and muscle twitching. Seizures are uncommon but can occur.

The benzodiazepines are prescription drugs. They are banned in specific sports by the USOC and IOC but not by the NCAA.

BETA BLOCKERS

Beta adrenergic blockers, or beta blockers, are relatively new drugs, which counter the effects of adrenalin and noradrenalin on the cardiovascular system. Beta blockers have a variety of medical uses including a role in treating hypertension, preventing migraine headaches, protecting against angina or chest pain, and helping to prevent cardiac rhythm problems.

The effects of the beta blockers are to reduce "beta" sympathetic tone, resulting in a decrease in heart rate, cardiac output, and resting blood pressure. These changes tend to be more dramatic during exercise when blood flow to all tissues except the brain is reduced.

Negative effects of the beta blockers include excessively slowed heart rate, congestive heart failure, hypotension (low blood pressure), and parasthesias (tingling, numbness). Lightheadedness, depression, and insomnia can also occur, as well as weakness, nausea, vomiting, cramps, diarrhea, and bronchial spasm (constriction of the smooth muscle of the lungs). In certain medical conditions, the use, and especially the termination of use, of beta blockers must be done very carefully. Toxic levels of the drug include some of the reactions already mentioned, especially slowed heart rate, cardiac failure, hypotension, and bronchial spasm.

Tolerance and addiction or withdrawal are not major problems with the beta blockers, compared to other drugs.

Because some beta blockers have been shown to reduce tremor, thus giving a "steadying effect," athletes have shown some interest in these drugs. Most of this interest has been in sports where a "steady hand" is important, such as in shooting and archery. Athletes in other sports where steadiness is important, such as ski jumping, dancing, and gymnastics, have also shown an interest in the drugs. However, there is no evidence that the use of beta blockers actually improves athletic performance. In addition, in normal athletes, or in those with uncomplicated hypertension, beta blockers impair endurance performance, especially if performance lasts over 30 minutes.

Beta blockers are prescription medications. They are banned by the USOC and IOC. They are banned by the NCAA for specific sports.

Table 8-8
Representative Beta Blockers

Generic Name	Trade Name
atenolol	Tenormin
metoprolol	Lopressor
nadolol	Corgard
pindolol	Visken
propranolol HCl	Inderal
timolol	Blocadren

BLOOD DOPING

Blood doping is the use of blood transfusions (intravenous injection of whole blood, packed red blood cells, or blood substitutes) to enhance performance. While blood transfusions have a place during surgery to replace blood loss and the like, blood doping has been used for athletic performance.

Blood doping usually involves removing one pint of the athlete's blood three to four weeks before a competitive event.

The packed red blood cells are frozen and stored under sterile conditions. The athlete's normal blood volume is restored during the continued training period. One to two days (24 to 48 hrs) prior to the competitive event, the athlete's blood is re-infused. This infusion of red blood cells increases the oxygen-carrying ability of the blood.

The desired effect of blood doping is to increase endurance through this increased oxygen-carrying capacity. It is similar in principle to high-altitude training, which is more difficult and costly to achieve.

Although blood doping has gained some popularity, the evidence regarding its results is conflicting. There are risks, including mismatched transfusions, infections, and clotting problems. The unpredictability of the effects of blood doping is illustrated by the 1984 Olympics, where seven members of the U.S. cycling team reportedly used blood doping. Among these athletes, four won medals, but three experienced flu-like symptoms and performed poorly.

Blood doping is obviously a technique that must be done under the supervision of a physician. The opinion of the American College of Sports Medicine can be summarized in this excerpt from its stand on blood doping as on ergogenic aid:

> It is the position of the American College of Sports Medicine that the use of blood doping as an ergogenic aid for athletic competition is unethical and unjustifiable, but that autologous RBC infusion is an acceptable procedure to induce erythrocythemia in clinically controlled conditions for the purpose of legitimate scientific inquiry.

According to the USOC/IOC, blood doping is prohibited and evidence confirming this practice is cause for a punitive action, comparable to that for using a banned substance. The NCAA also bans blood doping. Perhaps for this reason, athletes and physicians using this technique prefer to call it an array of other terms such as "boosting," "packing," or "supplementing," to try to reduce attention paid to it.

CAFFEINE (THEOPHYLLINE, THEOBROMINE)

The use of caffeine and the related substances, theophylline and theobromine, dates back to prehistoric man. These substances are found in many plants worldwide and since ancient times have been believed to have stimulant and mood-lifting properties. Among their medical uses is inclusion in many over-the-counter medications to help stay awake and stimulate, and in bronchial asthma and headache remedies. Caffeine is generally found in coffee, colas, tea, and cocoa. Theophylline is found mainly in tea, and theobromine in cocoa and such cocoa products as chocolate candy.

The effects of caffeine and the related substances are vasodilation and increased blood flow. There is an increase in resting heart rate, metabolism and burning of energy, urine production, and blood pressure. Appetite decreases, and the substances can irritate the bowel, leading to diarrhea or constipation.

Negative effects from long-term use are not clear, but it has been questioned whether caffeine and the related substances may have some relation to heart attacks and difficulties in pregnancy, and with developmental problems in newborns. If five to ten grams of caffeine are ingested, death may ensue. However, undesirable reactions have been observed following the ingestion of just one gram. These reactions include insomnia, restlessness, overexcitement, and a progression to mild delirium. There may be sensory disturbances, such as light flashes, ringing in the ears, and the like. There may be muscle tension and tremulousness, tachycardia (rapid heart rate), and extra heartbeats, cardiac arrhythmias, and seizures as well.

There is some suggestion that caffeine improves the racing performance of cross country skiers, especially at high altitudes, and may improve the capacity for muscular work in humans.

While caffeine and the related substances are legal, use of them beyond a certain amount is banned by the United States Olympic Committee. Amounts greater than 12 micrograms per milliliter of urine are considered illegal by the USOC. The NCAA uses a standard of 15 mcg/ml. Because of this, athletes need to be very careful about the amount of caffeine they ingest and also must be wary of preparations that may contain caffeine or the related substances (see Table 8-9). For example, two cups of coffee, four colas, one No-Doz, Empirin, or Anacin, will produce about three to six mcg of caffeine per milliliter of urine.

Table 8-9

Caffeine-Containing Over-the-Counter Drugs

I. Stimulants	II. Cold and Allergy Medications
Caffedrine capsules	Anodynos Forte
Double-E Alertness capsules	BC All Clear
No-Doz	Cenagesic Tablets
Prolamine capsules	Coryban-D Capsules
Quick Pep tablets	Dristan
Tirend capsules	Duradyne Forte Tablets
Vivarin tablets	Euphenex Tablets
	Fendol
	Hista-Compound No. 5
	Midran Decongestant
	Neo-Synephrine Compound
	Sinarest Tablets
	Super Anahist
	Triaminicin Tablets

COCAINE (AND CRACK)

Cocaine is the focus of much current attention in sports as well as society as a whole. Cocaine is a white crystalline alkaloid derived from the coca plant indigenous to South America. In its usual final form, cocaine is a white crystalline powder, cocaine hydrochloride. Cocaine is sniffed, swallowed, or injected for use. It can be smoked, as well, but only in its pure form, so that before it is smoked, the hydrochloride portion must be removed or "freed" by a process known a "free-basing." Cocaine is also known as coke, snow, and flake.

Cocaine has a very long history of use. Coca leaves and coca paste have been used as a stimulant by native Indian inhabitants of the Andes Mountains for almost 3,000 years. In its modern form, cocaine has been used since the 1850s.

Cocaine abuse has become a major societal concern. The National Institute on Drug Abuse estimates there are five to six million regular cocaine users in the United States. In the mid-1960s, the total worldwide production of cocaine was 500 kg per year (1100 pounds). This is estimated to be the average planeload today. The number of emergency room admissions due to cocaine use is up 500 percent over the last three years. Total annual cocaine-related deaths amount to 700 a year, a number that has tripled in the last three years.

Cocaine is a problem in sports, too, and not just at the professional level, where sale and use among players has made headlines. Consider the comments of a high school football player from south central Los Angeles:

> "You know how many people you run into who are dealing drugs? The ice cream truck comes by, I go out to buy a Popsicle and the driver says, 'I got a little more than ice cream here.'"[3]

Cocaine was used initially in medicine as a local anesthetic for eye surgery. This use was discontinued when it was found that corneal damage was a side effect. It does continue to have a role as an anesthetic and as a vasoconstrictor to reduce pain and bleeding during surgery of the upper respiratory tract or the nose.

As a stimulant, the main effect of cocaine use is increased motor activity. Unlike the use of amphetamines, cocaine use reduces aggressive behavior. Users experience less hunger and thirst and an increase in respiration, and heart rate, body temperature, and blood pressure.

The psychological effects of cocaine are influenced by the dose taken, setting in which it is taken, route of administration (how the drug is taken), and characteristics and experience of the user. In general, euphoria and a rush are experienced. There is a sense of increased mental alertness, sexual desire, and sensory awareness. The person feels more energetic and confident and is more talkative. As noted, appetite decreases and loss of sleep occurs.

Athletes may use cocaine either for recreational reasons or in hopes of enhancing performance.

With repeated use, the high may become unobtainable and can be replaced by feelings of anxiety, depression, and restlessness. Shortly after the first high, the crash occurs, which consists of sleepiness, irritability, depression, and a lack of motivation. When cocaine is smoked, the crash can occur within seconds of the original high. Users often increase the amount of cocaine used in the hope of regaining the high, but to no avail. Continually increasing dosages can lead to a variety of other problems.

Route of administration was mentioned as an important influence on the effect of the drug. The most common form of administration is nasally or snorting. When cocaine is snorted, there is an immediate numbing of the nose, followed by "the freeze," in which nothing occurs for approximately five minutes. A sense of gradually increasing and mild exhilaration, euphoria, and energy then occurs. The feeling peaks in 10 to 20 minutes and subsides within an hour. When cocaine is injected, the results are similar, but there is also the sensation of a rush that occurs within five minutes of the injection and subsides within a half-hour. Free-basing (smoking) is said to provide a rush as well as more intense feelings of vigor and pleasure.

It is unclear whether true tolerance occurs to cocaine effects. There is probably some tolerance to some of the physiological effects of the drug. There may be some tolerance to the subjective effects, although these apparently disappear rapidly with nonuse. Also, a reverse tolerance—increasing sensitivity with use—has been reported. Based on individual reports, rather than scientific evidence, however, it seems that repeated use makes it more difficult to get high.

Whether cocaine is addicting and whether there is a withdrawal syndrome is also unclear. It is difficult to separate withdrawal and dependency effects from those of chronic use.

Drugs: The Good and the Bad

However, because there is no reliable and clear-cut syndrome following the discontinuation of cocaine use, general medical opinion is that cocaine does not produce physical addiction in the usual sense. However, a variety of symptoms have been reported and can occur when cocaine use is stopped. These include depression, agitation, sweating, chills, social withdrawal, drug craving, and eating and sleeping disturbances. Unlike the case of true withdrawal, many of these effects do not abate when the drug is readministered.

Side effects and toxic effects of cocaine are pervasive. Vomiting can occur as cocaine stimulates the brain center controlling vomiting. High doses can produce tremors and convulsions. The central nervous system can collapse, leading to respiratory failure and cardiac arrest. Cocaine can increase certain types of seizures. In certain people, sudden cardiac death or stroke can occur. It is also important to note that some individuals lack a certain enzyme, which renders them unable to break down cocaine and eliminate it from the body. For these people, even a small dose can be lethal.

Cocaine psychosis is another potential side effect. This is a state of paranoia with delusions of persecution, and can involve visual and tactile hallucinations such as the sensation of insects crawling under the skin.

Regular users report other unpleasant side effects from the continued or chronic use of cocaine. These include fatigue, seizures, nausea, vomiting, chronic insomnia, severe headaches, nasal problems, reduced sexual performance, restlessness, irritability, attention and perceptual difficulties, depression, anxiety, loss of interest in friends and activities, and an inability to resist the drug when it is available.

There are also some indirect, but nevertheless important, dangers from cocaine use, as well. These include decreased job performance, interpersonal problems, and financial problems, due to the cost of the drug. Hepatitis and other infections can occur. Death or injury from car accidents, suicide from postuse depression, and burns from explosions from the chemicals used to prepare the cocaine (as reportedly happened to comedian Richard Pryor) can also occur. Finally, drug interactions are unpredictable, especially when drugs are mixed, as in a "speed ball" (heroin and cocaine), which is said to have accounted for the death of comedian John Belushi.

Crack is a form of cocaine that is now becoming widely available in the United States. It is considerably cheaper than traditional cocaine and is suitable for smoking. It is called crack because of the sound made by the crystals popping when they are heated. It is also known as rock, because of its appearance.

The effects and dangers described for cocaine apply to crack as well. However, crack *has* been reported to be addictive. In addition, because it is almost pure cocaine (not diluted or adulterated with other drugs) and is smoked, the effects are even more intense. Overdose is also more frequent and deaths have been reported. Crack is a widely available, relatively inexpensive, rapidly addicting form of cocaine that can cause overdosage and death.

Cocaine is a Schedule II drug, and tightly controlled. It is banned for use by the USOC and IOC, as well as the NCAA. There is a toll-free hotline available for questions or problems related to cocaine use: 1-800-COCAINE.

CORTICOSTEROIDS

The corticosteroid drugs derive from substances secreted by the adrenal cortex (the outer layer of the adrenal gland) in the body or they are synthetic models of these substances. Medically, they are used in the treatment of rheumatic and collagen diseases, dermatologic problems, allergy and respiratory problems.

The effects of the corticosteroid drugs are to reduce inflammation and pain. They are important drugs in some asthmatic conditions where they are given by inhalation. Athletes may abuse these drugs by relying on them rather than rehabilitation for injuries.

There are significant side effects to their use, including blood problems such as aplastic anemia, hypertension, peptic ulcer, encephalopathy (problems with brain function), and hepatitis. Other problems can include suppression of natural production of the body's steroids, muscle wasting, pain and weakness, delayed wound healing, and increased susceptibility to infection. There may be amenorrhea, nausea, vomiting, decreased appetite, problems with peptic ulcers, acne, and hirsutism (excessive hair growth).

Drugs: The Good and the Bad

Table 8-10
Representative Corticosteroids

Generic Name	Trade Name
beclomethasone dipropionate	Beclovent
betamethasone sodium phosphate	Celestone
cortisone	Cortisone, Cortone
dexamethasone	Baycadron Elixir
dexamethasone sodium phosphate	Ak-Dex, Bay-Dex, Dalalone, Decadron Phosphate, Hexadrol Phosphate, Savacort-D
flunisolide	Aerobid
hydrocortisone	Hydrocortisone
hydrocortisone acetate	Biosone, Cortef Acetate
methylprednisolone acetate	Bay-Mep 40, Medralone
prednisolone	Cortalone
prednisone	Cortan, Deltasone, Lid Pred, Meticorten, Orasone
triamcinolone	Aristocort
triamcinolone diacetate	Amcort, Aristocort Forte, Articulose-50, Cenocort Forte, Triamolone "40"

Withdrawal symptoms are noted with steroid use. These include anorexia, nausea, vomiting, headache, fever, joint pain, weight loss, and hypotension (low blood pressure).

The corticosteroid drugs require a prescription for use. The use of corticosteroids is banned by the USOC and IOC except for topical use, inhalational therapy, and local or intra-articular (in the joint) injections. Any team doctor wishing to administer such drugs intra-articularly or locally to a competitor must give written notification to the USOC or IOC Medical Commission. The oral, intramuscular, or intravenous use of corticosteroids is banned.

In the NCAA, use of corticosteroids must be declared and reasons and methods of use described in detail.

DIURETICS

Diuretics are another class of drugs abused by some athletes. The use of diuretics in medicine is to help eliminate fluid from the body and to help aid in the treatment of certain pathological conditions such as heart failure, kidney failure, or hypertension. However, diuretics are sometimes misused by athletes to accomplish two things. One is to reduce weight quickly

Table 8-11
Examples of Diuretic Drugs

Generic Name	Trade Name
acetazolamide	Diamox, AK-Zol, Dazamide
amiloride	Midamor
bendroflumethiazide	Naturetin
benzthiazide	Aquatag, Exna, Hydrex, Marazide, Proaqua
bumetanide	Bumex
chlorthalidone	Hygroton, Hylidone, Thalitone
diclofenamide	Daranide
furosemide	Lasix
hydrochlorothiazide	Esidrix, HydroDIURIL, Oretic, Thiuretic
spironolactone	Alatone, Aldactone
triamterene	Dyrenium

Drugs: The Good and the Bad

where weight categories are involved so that a competitor may gain an advantage by being placed in a different category. They are also used to attempt to reduce the concentration of drugs in the urine by promoting more rapid excretion of urine, as in cases where an individual wants to evade drug testing procedures.

The use of diuretics to effect rapid weight loss carries with it major health risks. Diuretics can raise cholesterol levels and can cause stomach distress, dizziness, blood problems, muscle spasms, and weakness. At toxic levels, lethargy and coma can occur. Attempts to reduce weight artificially in order to compete in a different weight class or to dilute urine to escape drug detection both represent manipulations that are unacceptable in sports on ethical grounds. Misuse of diuretics in sports also can lead to dehydration and heat-related problems. There is also the possibility of rapidly losing potassium, which can cause heart problems.

The USOC and IOC have banned the use of diuretics by athletes. The same is true for the NCAA.

DMSO

DMSO, dimethyl sulfoxide, probably falls most closely with the nonsteroidal anti-inflammatory drugs for categorization purposes. It is a liquid preparation alleged to have anti-inflammatory properties, and is used to treat interstitial cystitis. Some athletes believe that it relieves pain and discomfort when rubbed on an affected area, better than rest and heat do. Scientific confirmation of these effects seems to be lacking.

There are some negatives concerning the use of DMSO. First, human toxicity has not been established, although eye toxicity in animals has been reported. There is also concern about serum enzyme changes (disturbance of chemicals in the blood) and anemia. Second, DMSO produces a pungent breath odor. Finally, it is an excellent solvent and skin penetrant, which means that it can enable drugs and impurities to enter the system.

It is not marketed in the United States, nor has it been approved by the US Food and Drug Administration. DMSO is not banned, but it is not recommended by the USOC, IOC, or NCAA.

HUMAN GROWTH HORMONE

Human growth hormone (HGH) has attracted much attention in sports recently. While it is not a steroid, it is often used by athletes in an attempt to increase muscular strength. Secreted by the pituitary gland, this hormone helps to regulate growth. An alternative source of growth hormone is from animals, as only recently can enough HGH be made by recombinant DNA technology.

HGH is used medically to treat individuals whose growth is significantly delayed or retarded for a variety of reasons.

As suggested, athletes look to human growth hormone as a means to increase muscular strength. It may be used in conjunction with anabolic steroids. Sometimes HGH is used alone because it may be harder to detect in drug testing. However, there is no evidence that the use of HGH increases strength. In addition, nonhuman growth hormone is without physiological effect. One other approach used by athletes is to stimulate increased production of their own natural HGH. Various attempts at this have not been successful.

As with any drug or substance, excessive and inappropriate use can lead to problems. Human growth hormone can be related to the onset of diabetes. Further injection of HGH can reduce or neutralize endogenous or normally present growth hormone in an athlete's system.

HGH is banned as a related substance by the USOC and IOC. It is banned by the NCAA and any evidence confirming its use may be cause for punitive action.

INHALANTS

The use of inhalants or "sniffing" has gone through a variety of cycles and fads. People have experimented with sniffing substances ranging from gasoline to antiperspirant sprays. The first inhalants used to gain a high were anesthetic agents, such as chloroform, ether, and nitrous oxide. Some of these substances were believed to produce insight, wisdom, and mind expansion, similar to the hallucinogenic drugs that came later. Many lost their popularity when their toxic effects became apparent. While some inhalants of an anesthetic nature obviously have medical uses, most of the other products in which

Drugs: The Good and the Bad

Table 8-12
Representative Inhalants

Substance	Source
acetone	nail polish remover
benzene	adhesives, aerosols, degreasers, gasoline, glues, spray shoe polish
freon	aerosols
naptha	glues, lacquers, lighter fluids, paint removers
toluene	gasoline, glues, lacquers, paint removers

inhalants are found have domestic and industrial uses (see Table 8-12).

The effect of sniffing the inhalants is intoxication. Light-headedness, euphoria, ringing in the ears, double vision, staggering gait, and distorted motor movements result. There can be an unpleasant breath odor, an increase in salivation, and irritation to the eyes and nose.

Depending on the product used, toxic levels can create problems. Delusions, hallucinations, and mental confusion can occur. Individuals have been known to act out impulsive actions, such as trying to fly. Death from lack of oxygen can result from inhaling substances from plastic bags. Neurologic impairment and cardiac rhythm problems have been reported. Various levels of reduced breathing function can occur, including hypoxia (oxygen deficiency), as well permanent damage to the deep structures of the lungs.

Tolerance appears to occur with the inhalants. Chronic users require higher doses and more rapid delivery to achieve effects.

Addiction and withdrawal symptoms appear to be minimal. However, "feeling bad," fine tremors, irritability, and anxiety have been reported, and psychological dependence can occur.

Chronic effects of use range from mild to questionable problems with bone marrow depression, liver, kidney and brain damage.

Most inhalants are readily available or, if they are controlled, abuse of them is classified as a misdemeanor. However, concern over inhalant abuse is growing and some areas and jurisdictions have restricted the sale of items, such as airplane glue, to minors. Some corporations add additional chemicals to their products to produce nasal irritation and discomfort if the product is misused.

Inhalants are not specifically banned by the USOC, IOC, or NCAA. However, certain inhalants could be banned as related substances if their effects are similar to other illegal drugs.

LSD AND THE PSYCHEDELIC/HALLUCINOGENIC DRUGS

Psychedelic/hallucinogenic drugs are a group of drugs that alter perception and the state of consciousness. Representative psychedelic/hallucinogenic drugs are listed in Table 8-13. The best known is probably LSD. Some of the psychedelic/hallucinogenic drugs have a history dating at least as far back as the time of the Spanish conquest.

The peyote cactus (its derivative is mescaline) and certain mushrooms (its derivative is psilocin) are found in the southwestern United States and Mexico and their effects were well-known by the natives. LSD and its effects originally gained attention in 1943 because it was believed that they could be used to simulate mental illness for scientific study. In the 1960s, LSD became popular as a mind-expanding drug, which would facilitate self-exploration. The credo of "turn on, tune in, drop out" is ascribed to LSD advocates of that time.

The psychedelic/hallucinogenic drugs have been used for a variety of medical and therapeutic benefits, all of which have generally been abandoned because of a lack of evidence of their effectiveness and their negative side effects. At one time or another, however, these now-abandoned functions included uses as an aid in psychotherapy, as a model of mental illness, to induce tranquility and decrease the need for opiates, and as an aid in the treatment of cancer patients in the terminal stages of their disease. Their use by athletes is mainly for recreational and not performance-enhancing reasons.

Drugs: The Good and the Bad

Table 8-13
Representative Psychedelic/Hallucinogenic Drugs

Chemical Name	Common Name
diethyltryptamine	DET
dimethyltryptamine	DMT
lysergic acid diethylmide	LSD
	mescaline
	peyote
phencyclidine	PCP
	psilocybin
2,5,Dimethoxy-4-methylamphetamine (and, perhaps, various other compounds)	STP

The psychedelic/hallucinogenic drugs share many common characteristics, but there are also differences among them, depending on the specific substance. Also, as with some other categories of abused drugs, it is not always certain that the exact same compounds always exist under the same name. STP is a prime example: it has often been suspected that the term is applied to more than one substance or combination of compounds when it is sold and used on the street. Therefore, discussion of the effects of the psychedelic/hallucinogenic drugs will focus on the characteristics of LSD as representative for this group.

Physically, LSD produces increased heart rate, decreased blood pressure, decreased respiration, and dilation of the pupils. Hyperreflexia (overactive reflexes), tremor, nausea, muscular weakness, and increased body temperature can also occur, as well as dizziness, drowsiness, and paresthesias (numbness, tingling).

Certainly, the psychological effects of LSD are the most dramatic. LSD is a very powerful drug so that even minute amounts produce strong effects. The use of LSD heightens awareness of sensory input and produces the perception of enhanced sense of clarity, but also decreases control over what is experienced. Many users feel like passive observers of the environment rather than active participating forces. Time seems to be slowed; the environment is seen as novel, beautiful, and harmonious. Awareness turns inward, things seem more meaningful, the sense of truth becomes more obvious. The boundaries between objects or between the user and other objects can blur or dissolve totally. Wave-like perceptual changes and visual illusions are produced.

Among the negative effects of LSD, the "bad trip" is probably of most concern to LSD users. A bad trip brings panic and terror, and decreased control over experiences can be frightening, as can feelings of disintegration of the self.

Chronic use produces other negative effects, as well. Anxiety, paranoia, and psychoses have been described, as has brain damage. Flashbacks, or recurrences of the LSD experience without further ingestion of the drug, are reported in at least 15 percent of users. Prolonged depression can also be seen. The genetic effects of LSD use are unclear, but the drug should be avoided during pregnancy. Finally, despite the so-called "insights" and "mind expansion" reported by LSD users, there is little evidence of positive long-term changes in personality, beliefs, behavior, or attitudes.

Table 8-14
Representative Street Names for LSD

blue caps	pink dots
blue dots	purple flats
blue doubledomes	purple owsleys
brown caps	purple wedges
green caps	yellow caps
orange wedges	yellow dots
paisley caps	white lightning

Drugs: The Good and the Bad

Death from direct use of LSD is rare. However, death from accidents or acting out in relation to the psychological and perceptual changes has occurred. Tolerance to the behavioral effects of LSD is high and occurs rapidly. On the other hand, tolerance quickly disappears with nonuse. Withdrawal and addiction are not seen as a problem with LSD.

Clearly,the use of LSD and other hallucinogens is not likely to enhance athletic performance. And, indeed, maintaining a strict and disciplined training regimen can be very difficult when using these drugs.

The psychedelic/hallucinogens are generally listed as Schedule I drugs and, therefore, are illegal. They are not considered performance enhancers by the USOC. They are not banned by the USOC, IOC, or NCAA.

MARIJUANA

Marijuana is another drug with an extensive history. Its use is also widespread. Depending on where it is used, marijuana is known by various names—hashish, charas, bhang, ganja, and dagga. Common street names are pot, grass, and mary jane.

Marijuana does have potential usefulness in medicine. Its antinausea and relaxant effects have lead to its use in some cancer treatment programs. It also works to reduce pain and convulsions. A role has been suggested for marijuana in the treatment of glaucoma. While the medical use of marijuana is more prevalent in some other parts of the world, such use in the United States occurs only under special circumstances. Athletes may use marijuana to relax, either recreationally or (unwisely) to manage the stress of competition.

The physical effects of marijuana include an increase in systolic blood pressure (the highest pressure from a heart beat) and heart rate, sometimes 20 to 50 beats per minute. Too much pressure can cause a blood vessel to burst. Increases in body temperature and sweating occur. The noticeable increase in hunger that stems from marijuana use has been called "the munchies" by some users. Dry mouth and throat and reddening of the eyes (unrelated to smoke irritation) also can occur.

Marijuana also produces decreases in perception, attention, memory, and ability to process information. There is also a decline in the ability and motivation to do complex tasks. Aggressiveness lessens with use. Feelings of well-being and euphoria, as well as relaxation and sleepiness, are experienced. Individuals using marijuana have reported more vivid visual images and enhanced hearing. Time is distorted and seems to pass more slowly. A decrease in empathy in people using the marijuana has been reported. Other effects related to performance are discussed below. It is interesting to note that the setting and expectations often have a profound influence on the type and degree of effects that are experienced.

Toxic levels of marijuana can produce frank hallucinations (seeing things that don't exist), delusions, paranoia, or confused thinking. Anxiety up to levels of panic can occur. There can also be nausea and vomiting. Death by smoking excessive amounts of marijuana is not considered a problem.

Tolerance occurs to certain aspects, such as the cardiovascular effects. Interestingly, chronic users report a better "high" with more use—that is, a reverse tolerance.

Withdrawal and addiction are not part of the marijuana picture, although psychological addiction certainly can occur. In addition, individuals terminating marijuana use reported a variety of discomforts, including irritability, restlessness, nervousness, decreased appetite and weight loss, insomnia, tremor, chills, and increased body temperature.

The chronic use of marijuana has been related to decreased ovarian function and decreased sperm production. Bronchitis and asthma may be related to chronic smoking of the drug. A significant decrease in memory and motivation and an increase in apathy and dullness have been noted and named the "amotivational syndrome."

The effects of marijuana are such that sport performance detriments are more likely to occur than enhancements. A decrease in driving skills, even at minimal levels of use, has been demonstrated. In addition to this, and the effects already mentioned, marijuana decreases balance and stance stability, decreases muscle strength and hand steadiness, and at high levels can increase simple motor and reaction time. Despite this, a significant number of athletes report using marijuana.

Drugs: The Good and the Bad

Marijuana is a Schedule I drug and is illegal in the United States. It is currently not tested for by the USOC or IOC, unless requested by a national governing board.

Marijuana is banned by the NCAA. For marijuana/THC, this means a finding of the concentration of the THC metabolite in the urine in excess of 25 nanograms per milliliter.

METHAQUALONE

Methaqualone is one of the sedative/hypnotic drugs that has been abused extensively in recent years. During the 1950s methaqualone was found to have hypnotic properties. Despite indications of abuse potential from experience with its use in other countries, it was introduced in the United States in 1965 along with claims of low abuse potential. This has proven to be a mistake, as methaqualone has become one of the "most popular downers" on the black market. It has since been re-scheduled to level II—high abuse potential.

Medical uses for methaqualone are limited to use as an aid to help people sleep. However, it is no better than many other available and safer drugs. Methaqualone may be abused by athletes and others as a downer.

Physical and psychological effects are much like those of the barbiturates. Negative or side effects include nausea, weakness, and indigestion. There may be numbness and tingling. Rashes can occur. A feeling like that of a "hangover" is also seen with methaqualone. Chronic use of high doses can result in clumsiness, unsteadiness, impaired dexterity, defective judgment, and problems in concentrating.

Tolerance develops to methaqualone. Addiction with a clear withdrawal syndrome also occurs. Convulsions, tremors, delirium, nightmares, severe headache, and abdominal pain happen with abrupt termination of the drug. Death from overdose is also a possibility. Chances of death from overdose increase greatly (because much less of the drug is needed) if methaqualone is combined with other depressants, such as barbiturates, alcohol, or marijuana.

Several common misconceptions exist concerning methaqualone:

Methaqualone is an aphrodisiac.

Methaqualone is a safe downer since it is not a barbiturate.

Methaqualone is not addicting.

"Luding out" is safe and methaqualone can be used with alcohol.

None of these statements is true.

As noted, methaqualone is a Schedule II drug. It is banned in specific sports by the USOC and IOC; however, it is not on the banned list of the NCAA.

Table 8-15
Representative Trade Names for Methaqualone

Dimethacol	Quāālude
Optimil	Somnafac
Parest	Sopor

NARCOTIC ANALGESICS/OPIOIDS

The opioid drugs have been described and mentioned as early as the third century B.C. The drugs are derived from the poppy plant, and the term opium literally means "juice" (of the poppy). Opium smoking has been done throughout history in the Far East and the West. In the West, many artists and writers smoked opium in the eighteenth century. Morphine played a major role in medicine during the Civil War.

Heroin was derived from morphine in 1898. Early trials with this new derivation of morphine lead to the belief that it was useful in curing both opium and morphine addiction. In what is today a clear irony, this highly addicting drug was originally named heroin because of its anticipated "heroic" curative properties.

In medicine, the narcotic analgesics are crucial for control of pain. In fact, they have been called "God's own medicine" by the famous physician, Sir William Osler. Narcotics are also used to relieve cough and diarrhea, and as a pre-anesthetic medication to reduce anxiety and promote sleep.

The effects of the narcotic analgesics depend on the particular drug. While some of the medications in this group are mild in their effects, the following description of narcotic effects will refer to the more potent members of this category.

The term narcotic comes from the Greek word for stupor. Thus, the main effect of narcotic drugs is sedation. Pain is relieved, without the loss of consciousness at an appropriate level. The respiration centers and cough reflex are depressed which slows the heart rate. The drugs can also produce body warmth and heaviness in the limbs. Lowered blood pressure, constipation, nausea, vomiting, itching of the nose, and contraction of the pupils occur. Opioids also produce mental clouding; euphoria; reduced hunger, sex drive, activity, aggressiveness, and ability to concentrate; drowsiness; and apathy.

When heroin is abused, it is "mainlined" (injected) or "skin popped" (injected just below the skin). Users describe the sensation of a so-called kick. Abuse of narcotics quickly turns to avoiding withdrawal symptoms, rather than trying to regain the enjoyment of the high, because of the strong addictive property of the drug.

Toxic levels of the narcotics cause increasing depression, pinpoint pupils, slowed respiration, respiratory failure, flushing and cyanosis, and death.

Tolerance to the drugs develops, but not to effects on constipation and pupillary constriction.

Withdrawal and addiction are clear. The withdrawal syndrome consists of frequent yawning, goose flesh (also known as goose bumps), increased salivation, watery eyes, nausea and vomiting, abdominal muscle cramps, limb tremors (jerking), weight loss, anxiety, irritability, loss of appetite, dilated pupils, muscle spasms, occasional convulsions, and sometimes death. Going cold turkey (totally withdrawing from drug use all at once) creates significant physical stress on the body and is a very difficult process.

The chronic effects of opioid use include the occurrence of infection, such as venereal disease, tuberculosis, hepatitis, and pneumonia. Reduced motivation and social deterioration can occur. Illegal activity can evolve because of the need to get money to support the drug habit. Needle marks or "tracks"

develop along injection sites. Death from an accidental overdose is always a possibility.

While heroin is a Schedule I drug, other potent drugs in this
group are listed in Schedule II. These include drugs such as
morphine, codeine, and Percodan. The milder drugs in this
group, like Talwin and Darvon, are Schedule IV drugs. The
USOC and IOC banned drug list includes these milder narcotic
analgesics, like Darvon and Talwin, among all opioids and
narcotics. The NCAA also bans use of these drugs in sport.
Athletes need to be especially careful when using medicine
that may contain some of these substances as part of their
formula, such as cough medicines like Cheracol and Romilar
(which contain codeine). Dextromethorphan is not banned.

Table 8-16
Representative Narcotic Analgesics

Generic Name	Trade Name or Source
codeine	found in Cheracol, Romilar
dextromethorphan	found in Dristan Ultra Colds Formula, Triaminic DM Colds Formula
diphenoxylate HCl	Lomotil
heroin (also known as H, horse)	
hydromorphone HCl	Dilaudid
meperidine	Demerol
methadone	Dolophine
morphine	
oxycodone	Percodan
papaverine	Pavabid
pentazocine HCl	Talwin
propoxyphene	Darvon

NICOTINE AND TOBACCO

The use of tobacco, like the other drugs discussed, has a long history. Nicotine, one of the most important components in tobacco, was first isolated from tobacco in 1828. There are no generally accepted medical uses for nicotine, although nicotine chewing gum is marketed to help reduce nicotine addiction caused by smoking.

Nicotine is a stimulant. Depending on how it is ingested, nicotine has various effects on the body. Smoking allows for transit of nicotine to the brain within seconds. The effect of nicotine is to increase heart rate and increase blood pressure. Nicotine inhibits stomach contractions, produces tremors, and decreases skin temperature. In novice smokers, nausea, vomiting, headache, and other unpleasant side effects are common.

Smoking produces more than just the ingestion of nicotine, however. Carbon monoxide is another substance ingested when tobacco is smoked. Carbon monoxide gas readily replaces oxygen in the blood, leading to decreased oxygen-carrying capacity. Many other substances are derived from smoking tobacco, including some that are carcinogenic (cancer-producing). Some of the other by-products of tobacco include ammonia, formaldehyde, creosote, phenols, and arsenic (derived from the fertilizers and insecticides used on the tobacco).

Tolerance develops to the side effects—headache, nausea, etc.—with repeated use. The body also appears to have an affinity for a certain level of nicotine. When this level drops because of abstention from smoking, the smoker often feels the "need" for another cigarette. Smokers then continue smoking until this level is achieved again. This is why smokers who change to low nicotine cigarettes often end up smoking more cigarettes—to maintain their same levels of nicotine.

Acute toxic effects do occur. Generally these include nausea, vomiting, dizziness, and weakness. Severe nicotine poisoning can result in convulsions, unconsciousness, and even death. The fatal dose of nicotine is about 16 mg.

The need for smokers to maintain a certain level of nicotine in the body should suggest that addiction to tobacco/nicotine occurs very readily. It can be very strong with significant withdrawal symptoms that make quitting smoking so difficult.

Symptoms of withdrawal from tobacco/nicotine include irritability, impatience, anxiety, headache, difficulty in concentrating, drowsiness or insomnia, cramps, hunger, tremors, and fatigue.

The long-term effects of smoking on health are very clear and well-publicized. Smoking is such a threat to health and is involved in so much disease and illness, that quitting smoking has been called the single most effective action a person can take to improve his health. Never starting to smoke is probably the smartest move a person, and especially an athlete, can make.

Smoking is related to heart disease, stroke, and peripheral vascular disease, as well as heartbeat irregularities and sudden death. It is a major contributor to lung cancer and other cancers, such as those of the mouth, larynx, and esophagus. Cancer in many other parts of the body is believed to be related to smoking, as well. Chronic obstructive pulmonary diseases, such as emphysema and chronic bronchitis, are related to smoking. Decreased birth weight in infants and increased spontaneous abortions in women who smoke have been reported.

It is important to realize that indirect smoke is also far from risk-free. Evidence also now exists to show that nonsmokers are affected by inhaling the smoke from smokers. These effects are both short-term and long-term.

Smokeless tobacco—chewing tobacco and snuff—deserve special mention because they are often associated with sports, especially baseball. The sight of a baseball player "chawing" tobacco and then spitting it is classic. Although many athletes think it must be healthier to use smokeless tobacco, it is not. Using this type of tobacco carries with it many risks.

A well-known example of young athletes wanting to emulate the professionals is that of an Oklahoma track star. He reportedly started using smokeless tobacco at the age of 11 or 12 because he saw his sports heroes using it. He died at 19 from a cancer that had spread from his tongue to his neck. It was his doctor's opinion that the smokeless tobacco has caused his cancer and subsequent death.

Babe Ruth was known as a tobacco chewer and heavy snuff user. Many people remember the typical image of the "Babe," with his robust and stocky build, standing at the plate, chewing his tobacco. However, he developed oral cancer and, at his death, weighed 137 pounds.

Although nicotine was often given and found in the urine or saliva of racehorses in the 1950s and early '60s, there is no reason to believe that human athletic performance is enhanced. Certainly, smoking stands to decrease conditioning and performance, if not disease.

Tobacco and nicotine, of course, are widely available. Nicotine is not on the USOC's or IOC's list of banned drugs. It is not banned by the NCAA. However, the NCAA is concerned about tobacco use, including smokeless tobacco, by its athletes. Therefore drug screening for nicotine may be conducted for research and nonpunitive purposes.

NONSTEROIDAL ANTI-INFLAMMATORY DRUGS
Nonsteroidal anti-inflammatory drugs (NSAIDS) are recently developed medications that are used to ease pain and inflammation of the muscles and joints. They are useful in musculoskeletal disorders and injuries, such as rotator cuff tendonitis (inflammation of the shoulder tendons) and breast stroker's knee in swimmers.

The effect of the NSAIDS is to relieve pain and to reduce inflammation, swelling, and fever.

There are side effects to the NSAIDS, which include dyspepsia, gastrointestinal bleeding, blood problems, and sedation.

Table 8-17
Representative Nonsteroidal Anti-Inflammatory Drugs

Generic Name	Trade Name
acetylsalicylic acid	aspirin
ibuprofen	Advil, Motrin, Nuprin
indomethacin	Indocin
naproxen	Naprosyn
phenylbutazone	Butazolidin

They also can interfere with the body's ability to regulate temperature and can predispose athletes to heat-related illness. Toxic levels of the drug can cause headache, nausea, depression, anemia, leukopenia, aplastic anemia, thrombocytopenia, and agranulocytosis (changes in blood cells). Butazolidin, once used widely, especially in sports, has fallen in disfavor because of its hematologic (blood) side effects and liver toxicity.

Addiction is not a problem with the NSAIDS. However, the danger posed by the NSAIDS is that athletes will use them without the supervision of a physician. This puts the athlete at risk of developing the above side effects. More likely, however, athletes abuse NSAIDS to compete when they should be resting and healing their injury. This is likely to cause a more serious and perhaps permanent injury, which could adversely affect an entire career.

NSAIDS generally require a prescription for use. In lower doses, some of the NSAIDS are now available in over-the-counter drugs. They are not on the USOC's, IOC's, or NCAA's list of banned drugs.

PHENCYCLIDINE

Phencyclidine, one of the psychedelic-hallucinogenic drugs, deserves special mention because of its popularity and profound effects. Phencyclidine was developed in the 1950s and first used as an anesthetic in animals and humans. This medical use was discontinued because of problems with delirium occurring in patients after anesthesia. In the early 1970s, phencyclidine was becoming a more popular abused drug taken by smoking or snorting. By the mid-1970s, it was widely abused and the focus of much concern. Phencyclidine is known by a variety of street names (see Table 8-18). Athletes may abuse phencyclidine for recreational purposes.

Phencyclidine produces a sense of intoxication with a staggering gait, slurred speech, nystagmus (eye movements related to dizziness) and numbness of the extremities. Sweating and muscular rigidity can occur. Psychologically, there is a change in body image, disorganized thinking, and apathy, and hostility and bizarre behavior can occur. Amnesia about such episodes is often present.

At higher levels, there is a noticeable increase in heart rate, blood pressure, and salivation. Sweating, fever, and repetitive movements are present. Toxic levels can also lead to psychotic states, violent behavior, and accidents. Psychoses can last weeks, even after a single dose. Convulsions, stupor, coma, and death are also possible.

Tolerance has been reported to some of phencyclidine's effects. It is difficult to separate the effects of chronic use from what may be withdrawal symptoms. On termination, complaints of craving for phencyclidine have been reported. Difficulties with memory, speech, and thinking have been noted and described as lasting six months to a year after use has stopped. Social withdrawal, isolation, anxiety, and severe depression are also seen with termination.

Phencyclidine is illegal. It is not considered a performance enhancer by the USOC, however, it is banned for some sports by the USOC and IOC. It is not listed as a banned substance by the NCAA.

Table 8-18
Street Terms for Phencyclidine

angel dust	mint weed
crystal	mist
cyclones	monkey dust
embalming fluid	PCP
elephant tranquilizer	peace pill
goon	rocket fuel
horse tranquilizer	scuffle
killer weed	super weed
KW	surfer

STRYCHNINE
Strychnine, a central nervous system stimulant, has been popular among athletics. It comes from the seeds of a tree native to India and was introduced into Germany in the sixteenth century as a rat poison. It is still used for this and accounts for many accidental poisonings. Medical uses for strychnine are essentially now nonexistent. It is often used to adulterate

street drugs. Athletes may hope for an increase in wakefulness and better reflexes from its use.

As a central nervous stimulant, it shares many of the effects of other stimulants and also acts as a convulsant.

Negative and toxic effects include stiffening of the face and neck muscles and an increased reflex excitability, where any sensory stimulus can lead to violent motor responses. There may be convulsions, and respiration can cease due to contractions of the diaphragm. Contractions of the thoracic and abdominal muscles can be very painful and can be followed by death.

Consequently, it is not surprising that, because of its dangerous properties, strychnine has lost popularity as a performance-enhancing drug.

Strychnine is banned by the USOC, IOC, and NCAA.

SYMPATHOMIMETIC DRUGS

Sympathomimetic drugs are chemically related to amphetamines. They occur naturally in several types of plants around the world, and were used in China for 2,000 years before their introduction to American medicine in the 1920s.

There are a variety of medical uses for the sympathomimetic drugs. They are used as nasal decongestants and for mild cases of asthma and bronchospasm, as well as to control hemorrhage, in hypotension, and to dilate the pupil of the eye. The sympathomimetics are also found in a variety of over-the-counter medications, such as cold remedies (see Table 8-19) and appetite suppressants.

The sympathomimetics are stimulants, therefore they increase blood pressure and cardiac output. Coronary and cerebral blood flow may be increased, as may flow to the muscles, but the heart's demand for oxygen also increases. There is some bronchial muscle relaxation as well.

Side effects tend to be rare, especially when the drugs are used in recommended doses. However, palpitations, nervousness, and undesired blood pressure increases can occur.

Toxic effects are rare, but include insomnia. An infrequent effect can be an amphetamine-like psychosis. Addiction or withdrawal is not a problem. However, overuse of these drugs can lead to rebound congestion (congestion that is made worse when the drug is stopped).

In the 1950s and '60s, it was suggested that sympathomimetics could enhance athletic performance. However, more recent studies show no marked effects.

Sympathomimetics are Schedule IV drugs and, therefore, require a prescription. However, as noted, they may be found

---

Table 8-19

Representative Sympathomimetic Drugs Found in Over-the-Counter Preparations

Generic Name	Over-the-Counter Preparation Source
ephedrine	Bronchotabs, Bronkaid, Nyquil, Quiet-Nite, Primatene
oxymetazoline HCl	AFRIN
phenylpropanolamine HCl	Allerest, Allergesic, Appedrine, Baer Decongestant C3 Capsules, Coricidin D, Day Care, Dexatrim, Halls, Novahistine DH, Novahistine Elixir, Ornacol capsules and liquid, Ornex, Prolamine, Robitussin-CF, Romilar 3, Romilar capsules, Sine-Off, Sinurex, Sinutab, TRIAMINIC, Vicks Formula 44
propylhexedrine	Benzedrex Inhaler
pseudoephedrine HCl	CHLOR-TRIMETON Decongestant Co-Tylenol, Novafed, Novafed A, Novahistine DMX, Robitussin-PE, SUDAFED
tetrahydrozoline HCl	Visine Eye Drops

in certain over-the-counter preparations in lower doses. They are on the USOC/IOC's banned list. They are banned by the NCAA. So, as with other drugs, it is important that athletes do not inadvertently ingest the drug. A classic example of this is the case of Rick DeMont, who was forced to return the gold medal that he won in swimming in 1972 because he tested positive for a sympathomimetic he used for the treatment of his asthma.

Inadvertent ingestion is a good likelihood because of the prevalence of these drugs in other preparations. It is important to read the label of any medication that you use. Table 8-20 lists sources of sympathomimetic found in over-the-counter drugs that are acceptable to the IOC.

Table 8-20

Representative Sympathomimetics Acceptable to the International Olympic Committee

Generic Name	Source
salbutamol	Proventil, Ventolin, Albuterol
terbutaline	Brethaine, Brethine, Bricanyl

VITAMINS

Vitamins are not exactly in the same category as the other drugs discussed here, but they need to be included because some athletes believe in their value and use them excessively. Vitamins are organic substances that must be provided in small quantities in the diet for the synthesis, by the tissues, of elements that are essential for metabolic functions.

While it is true that vitamin *deficiencies* can hurt athletic performance and health in general, there is no evidence that large doses can enhance athletic performance. However, many myths do exist, such as the belief that vitamin E enhances not only athletic performance, but sexual performance as well.

It is important to realize that while vitamin toxicity is rare, negative effects can occur from taking too much of a vitamin. For example, excessively high doses of vitamin A can lead to musculoskeletal pain, abnormal liver function, and elevated

Drugs: The Good and the Bad

plasma triglycerides (high amounts of certain kinds of fats in the blood).

The major side effect from excessive vitamin use continues to be wasted money. It has been said that Americans may have the most valuable urine in the world because of the amounts of vitamins they excrete, due to an erroneous belief in the beneficial effect of large doses. The role of megadoses of vitamins in sport has been summarized this way:

> The vitamin hoax is a crutch upon which many athletes lean, especially when their performance is below that which they hope to attain.[4]

Nutrition and adequate vitamin intake are essential for optimal athletic performance. However, just as in other areas of sports training, athletes should seek expert advice and should be cautious about fad diets or nutritional miracles.

Vitamins are not banned by the USOC, IOC, or NCAA. However, some so-called vitamin preparations sold in health food stores may contain banned substances as part of their ingredients.

VITAMIN B$_{15}$

Vitamin B$_{15}$ is a substance that deserves special mention because of unusual claims about its properties. It has been suggested that vitamin B$_{15}$ detoxifies toxic products in the human system. Among other claims, it supposedly can be used to prevent or treat cancer, heart disease, schizophrenia, allergies, diabetes, and glaucoma. It has been said to be helpful in slowing the aging process, as well as purifying air.

Vitamin B$_{15}$ is not a vitamin, however. It is pangamic acid, a food additive isolated from apricot kernels. The US Food and Drug Administration has indicated that it is not a vitamin or a pro-vitamin; that there is no accepted scientific evidence establishing nutritional properties; and that it has no medical, nutritional, or other usefulness. It is also suspected that many different substances go under the name of vitamin B$_{15}$.

Because of this lack of proof of a standard chemical entity and any evidence for its safe use or any benefit, Canada's

Food and Drug Directorate has banned the substance. Vitamin B$_{15}$ is not recommended for use, although it is not banned, by the USOC, IOC, or NCAA.

Table 8-21

Regulatory Status of Drugs by the USOC, IOC, and NCAA

DRUG	USOC/IOC	NCAA
alcohol	NOT banned, but may be tested for on request	banned for specific sports: riflery
amphetamines	banned	banned
anabolic steroids	banned	banned
antidepressants	banned for specific sports: biathlon, modern pentathlon	NOT banned
antipsychotics/ major tranquilizers	banned for specific sports: biathlon, modern pentathlon	NOT banned
barbiturates/sedatives/ hypnotics	banned for specific sports: biathlon, modern pentathlon	NOT banned
benzodiazepines	banned for specific sports: biathlon, modern pentathlon	NOT banned
beta blockers	banned	banned for specific sports: riflery
blood doping	banned	banned
caffeine	banned if urine concentration exceeds 12 mcg/ml	banned if urine concentration exceeds 15 mcg/ml
cocaine/crack	banned	banned
corticosteroids	oral, IM, IV banned; topical use okay; intra-articular use requires notification	use must be declared

DRUG	USOC/IOC	NCAA
diuretics	banned	banned
DMSO	NOT banned, not recommended	NOT banned
human growth hormone	banned	banned
inhalants	NOT banned	NOT banned
LSD/hallucinogens	banned	banned
marijuana	NOT banned; may be tested for on request	banned; test for urine concentration greater than 25 nanogram/ml
methaqualone	banned for specific sports: biathlon, modern pentathlon	NOT banned
narcotics/opioids	banned	banned
NSAIDS	NOT banned	NOT banned
nicotine/tobacco	NOT banned	NOT banned; may be tested for research purposes
phencyclidine (PCP)	banned for specific sports: biathlon, modern pentathlon	NOT banned
strychnine	banned	banned
sympathomimetics	banned	banned
vitamins	NOT banned, but some preparations may contain banned substances	NOT banned
vitamin B_{15}	NOT banned, not recommended	NOT banned

Chapter Nine

Saying No to Drugs:
SOME SUGGESTIONS

Saying No to Drugs

SOME SUGGESTIONS If you have read this far, you are now aware that drug abuse is an important and complex issue for sports and athletes. You may have known that before you read this book; however, perhaps it wasn't clear just how complicated, important, and pervasive the problem is.

Mastering the skills to say no to drugs in sports—for you to say no to drugs in your sport—is just as difficult as mastering the skills of your sport itself. Because the drug problem is so present, pervasive, and persuasive, saying no requires developing psychological and behavioral skills just the same as sports performance does. It will take time, effort, and practice, and it will not come easy. But you know that because you are an athlete, and as an athlete you know that success requires much effort.

Success in sports, and in saying no to drug abuse in sports, also requires a good strategy. This section of the book provides such a strategy to help you begin to develop skills to make your own independent decisions about drug use. Five approaches are presented here to help you.

The first strategy is assessing if you have the basic skills to make an independent decision about drug use. Next, you need a good game plan—knowing your values about sports and life. Third, a good defense is always necessary—strengthening your coping abilities. Fourth, success is impossible without a good offense—understanding the purpose of drug use and effective alternatives to such use. Finally, winning the big ones requires practice—using your skills to succeed in making your choice independently.

You can develop these skills by working through the exercises in the next section by yourself. If you prefer you can train with a friend or a group of friends instead. Sharing ideas and strategies is always a good method. Perhaps the best approach is to run through the training exercises by yourself and then check and share your results with other athletes, teammates, and close friends.

Some Basic Skills: Am I Ready to Decide?

Just as basic skills mastery is required for your sport before you can turn in an elite performance, some basic skills are required before you can successfully make an independent decision about drug use. To help assess your readiness to make such a decision, some pertinent basic skills are presented below. For each of the skills you should reflect seriously and evaluate how well you have mastered them and indicate this by circling the appropriate number on the decision line.

1 How willing am I to recognize drug use as a serious problem for sports?

1	2	3	4	5	6	7	8	9	10

What a bunch of garbage.

It is a major issue that sports and athletes must deal with it.

2 How willing am I to recognize drug use as a potential problem for all athletes including myself?

1	2	3	4	5	6	7	8	9	10

Hey, not my problem.

I need to work just as hard as any other athlete to make independent decisions on this matter.

3 How thoroughly have I read and understood the drug/ doping regulations for my sport?

1	2	3	4	5	6	7	8	9	10

Who cares?

I read and under-
stand all I can, but
if there's more in-
formation I want
that too.

4 How well do I understand the drug control measures used in my sport?

1	2	3	4	5	6	7	8	9	10

What for?

I understand them
and they mean
business.

5 How well do I understand the consequences of breaking the drug rules for my sport?

1	2	3	4	5	6	7	8	9	10

Why? I'd never
get caught.

Loud and clear.

6 How thorough have I been in gathering and reading information on the effects of drugs?

1	2	3	4	5	6	7	8	9	10

I knew it already.

I found all I could
but I can always use
more information.

7 How well can I evaluate whether information from a given source about drugs is reliable and true?

1	2	3	4	5	6	7	8	9	10

If I agree with it,
then it's true.

I know how to
evaluate whether
information is
based on good
scientific research
or it's just an opinion.

8 How well do I understand legitimate uses of each drug in question?

1	2	3	4	5	6	7	8	9	10

No need to be-
cause I'm going
use the drug for
my own purposes.

I can name at
least one medical
use for each drug.

9 How well do I understand the potential dangers of each drug in question?

1	2	3	4	5	6	7	8	9	10

Don't need to
know because it
won't happen to
me.

I can name at
least two dangers
for each drug.

10 How well do I understand the potential effect of drug abuse on my sports career?

1	2	3	4	5	6	7	8	9	10

I haven't thought
about it.

I've given it very
serious thought.

11 How well do I understand the potential effects of drug abuse on my personal life?

1	2	3	4	5	6	7	8	9	10

Sports are all that
counts.

I have an impor-
tant life outside of
sports that can be
seriously affected
by drug use.

12 How well do I understand the potential effects of drug abuse on my team?

1	2	3	4	5	6	7	8	9	10

I'm looking out for number one (me) only.

I have seriously considered how it might harm the team.

13 How well do I understand the legal consequences of drug use?

1	2	3	4	5	6	7	8	9	10

I'll never get caught.

I understand the implications for both sport and my personal life.

14 How willing am I to put forth the effort to learn to make a rational and independent decision about drug use in my sport?

1	2	3	4	5	6	7	8	9	10

I've got more important things to do.

It's worth whatever effort it takes.

15 How willing am I to help another teammate or athlete with his drug abuse issues?

1	2	3	4	5	6	7	8	9	10

Let him get his own help.

This is an issue that all athletes share and I'm glad to help.

How Ready Are You: How Good Are Your Basic Skills?

You can see how developed your basic skills are by looking at your score on the items you just completed. There are two ways to determine how prepared you are.

First, look at your score for each question. The chart below tells you what your score for each item means. Any score of 6 or below suggests a weakness.

SCORE	MEANING
0–2	You didn't make the cut.
3–6	You're on the bench.
7–10	You're ready to start.

Next add up your ratings for all the items together, then check what your overall score means by referring to the chart below. Any score below 125 suggests some deficits.

SCORE	MEANING
0–45	Novice
46–104	Amateur
105–125	Rookie
125–150	Elite/Professional

For those areas where you have deficits, you should get started on planning how to remedy and improve them. You can use the chart below to help you plan how to improve your basic skills in a given area and then follow through on it.

	Skill Area Deficit	How to Improve It
1	_____	_____
2	_____	_____
3	_____	_____
4	_____	_____
5	_____	_____

Saying No to Drugs

6 _____ _____

7 _____ _____

8 _____ _____

A Clear Game Plan: Values—What I Care About; Who Cares About Me

No game can be played or competition performed successfully without a strategy or plan. In sports and life, and especially in relation to drug use, an important part of the plan is recognition of your own values. You need to recognize those things that are important to you, that have meaning for you, that you are willing to work for. A clear game plan based on your own values helps to give you direction.

Athletes often do not take the time to assess their own values. They are too busy training and working hard to take time to reflect on the importance of things to them. Yet, doing so can add an important dimension to both your sport and your personal life.

Consider the comments of three-time Olympic biathlon competitor Lyle Nelson on the importance of values to athletes:

> This is an alarming statement, but I don't think most Americans are sure of their value system. It is perhaps our greatest cultural woe. You can only guess at your best course of action if you do not fully know your values. I don't mean just having a general understanding of what you admire. Let me give you an example. What is the most important thing in your life? What is second? And third? The answers should be automatic. To best achieve the things important to us, they should be well defined and conceived. If you haven't already done so, I strongly encourage you to take 10 minutes and prioritize your highest values. It's hard to stand tall when you are not sure what you stand for.

> I know that I could not properly coach you
> without an insight into your values, and I
> don't think you can adequately coach your-
> self without it either.[1]

Let's first look at your sports values. From the list that follows, number in order of importance to you, the various aspects of sports and competition in the spaces provided. If there are some aspects of sports that are important to you that are not listed, add them to the list and place them in order as well. If some from the list do not apply, you can omit them. For the time being, simply ignore the columns marked F and H. Place the number 1 next to the value that is most important to you. Place the number 2 next to the second most important value, and so on, until you have numbered all of the values important to you.

Potential Values of Sport	Order of Importance to Me	F	H
1 Winning and being the best	_____	_____	_____
2 Having fun	_____	_____	_____
3 Developing playing skills	_____	_____	_____
4 Traveling	_____	_____	_____
5 Making friends on the team	_____	_____	_____
6 Learning about the sport	_____	_____	_____
7 Developing my own health	_____	_____	_____
8 Developing psychological skills	_____	_____	_____
9 Striving to do my personal best	_____	_____	_____
10 Making others proud of me	_____	_____	_____
11 Being admired by others	_____	_____	_____
12 Making it to the pros or elite levels	_____	_____	_____
13 Getting money from sports	_____	_____	_____
14 Helping others with their performance	_____	_____	_____
15 Self-respect	_____	_____	_____
16 Setting and achieving goals	_____	_____	_____
17 Self-confidence	_____	_____	_____
18 Other	_____	_____	_____

Next is a list of things that are potentially important to you in your personal life, including sports participation. Once again, you should place these in their order of importance to you in the spaces provided. If there are some values that are important to you that have not been listed, add them and place them in order as well. If some values that are on the list do not apply to you, they can be omitted. Once again, ignore columns F and H for now.

Potential Personal Values	Order of Importance to Me	F	H
1 Having a good friend	_____	_____	_____
2 Family	_____	_____	_____
3 Sport	_____	_____	_____
4 School/work	_____	_____	_____
5 Having lots of friends	_____	_____	_____
6 Future careers/job	_____	_____	_____
7 Excitement	_____	_____	_____
8 Comfort	_____	_____	_____
9 Money	_____	_____	_____
10 Sense of accomplishment	_____	_____	_____
11 Social recognition	_____	_____	_____
12 Happiness	_____	_____	_____
13 Contentment	_____	_____	_____
14 Caring for someone else	_____	_____	_____
15 Having someone special care for me	_____	_____	_____
16 Being smart	_____	_____	_____

Potential Values of Sport	Order of Importance to Me	F	H
17 Being attractive	_____	_____	_____
18 Parties	_____	_____	_____
19 Religion/spiritual issues	_____	_____	_____
20 Being creative	_____	_____	_____
21 Sense of self-worth	_____	_____	_____
22 Other	_____	_____	_____

It is hoped that this exercise will have helped you think more clearly about what things are important to you and how important they are. One of the interesting things to see is where you place sports on your list of personal values. Also of importance is seeing where you placed winning as one of the values in sports.

Since athletes often rationalize drug use and abuse as evidencing their commitment to sports and their dedication to being number one, it is important to see where these values fall for you. If they are not number one on both of your lists, you may wonder why drug use to achieve a secondary goal would enter into consideration at all.

Even if sports and winning are at the top of your list, there is another question you should ask in relation to drug use: not how well drugs will help you achieve this goal (assuming they can) but How could drug use Foul up these values for you.

Whatever the ranking of your values on these lists, this is a good time to ask how drugs might foul up any of the values you just ranked; drug use can affect both your sports and your personal life.

You can now complete columns F and H. Under column F indicate for each value whether drugs could foul up this value for you and how easily this could happen. You can indicate this by giving each value an F rating:

1 Place one F if drugs could foul up this value and there is *some* likelihood that it could happen to you.

2 Place two F's if drugs could foul up this value and there is a *good* likelihood that it could happen to you.

3 Place three F's if drugs could foul up this value and it is *highly* likely this would happen to you.

4 Leave the space blank if drugs could not affect this value.

In the H column outline your thoughts on how drugs could foul up this value for you. Obviously the higher the F rating, the more serious the How column should be.

You now have an indication of what is important to you in sports and life. You also have a description of how these things can be lost by drug use. It is well to keep this in mind, especially the values with the triple F (FFF) rating. They are the real losses they could make you the real loser.

A Good Defense: Assessing Coping Strengths

All of us need ways to deal with things that challenge, confuse, or trouble us. The ways we use to deal with such things are called our coping mechanisms. There are many different ways of coping. Some ways of coping work better than others and some ways work better for some people than for others.

Coping resources are both external (outside of us) and internal (within us). Both types are important.

I. External Sources of Support

Complete the following questions. This will help you assess your external coping resources and abilities. Answer each in regard to drug use potential in your sport.

1 Who is (are) the person(s) I can go to for advice when I am confused?*

_____

_____

_____

*You can use the same person(s) to answer more than one question.

2 Who is (are) the person(s) I trust enough to share my concerns with?

_____

_____

_____

3   Who is (are) the person(s) I respect enough to listen to?

_____

_____

_____

4   Who is (are) the person(s) who care enough about me to be honest, fair, and concerned?

_____

_____

_____

5   Who is (are) the person(s) who keep(s) trying to put pressure on me to do things I don't feel right doing or want to do, even when I explain this to him(them)?

_____

_____

_____

What does this all mean? If you do not have names to answer questions 1 through 4, it is important to ask yourself why this is and how you can find some people to fill these roles and help you at these times. Question 5 is important, because persons whose names appear here should not be considered as resources for support; they are probably not acting in your best interest. The best people to go to for support to help you with your drug decision process are those whose names appear at least once in questions 1, 2, 3, or 4. The best person(s) to use as a resource is someone whose name appears in more than one answer. He or she obviously has a variety of attributes that are important to you.

II. Internal Support and Coping Mechanisms

Below are ways some people deal with problems, disappointments, and challenges. From the list, rank the ones you use in spaces provided in order of most used to least used. If some other ways of dealing with things that are important to you are not listed, add them and place them in order, as well. If some ways of coping from the list do not apply to you, they can be omitted.

Ways of Coping   **Order of Use**

DENIAL: I pretend it doesn't really exist.   _____

PROBLEM SOLVE: I try to find a way to fix or handle it step by step by planning and executing the plan.   _____

INFORMATION SEEK: I try to find out as much as I can about the problem to help me make a decision.   _____

AVOID: I do anything I can to avoid facing it.   _____

MINIMIZE: I pretend it is less of a problem than it really is.   _____

SHARE: I discuss my thoughts and feelings with others who are close to me and whom I trust.   _____

LAUGH IT OFF: I just make a big joke out of it and do not face it at all.   _____

GIVE UP: I give in and feel bad about it.   _____

BLAME OTHERS: I always try to make it look like someone else's fault or problem.   _____

BLAME MYSELF: I always take the blame and see it as my fault, even if that is not the case.   _____

USE HUMOR: I face the problem but use humor to lighten it up just a little.   _____

DEFER: I ask an authority what to do and then do whatever that person tells me.   _____

Ways of Coping   **Frequency**

FIND POSITIVES: I try to find something good
or positive in the situation.   _____

LEARN FROM IT: I try to find something I can
use the next time or in a similar situation, no
matter how bad the current situation might be.   _____

CATASTROPHIZE: I think of everything that
could go wrong in the situation or could make
things worse.   _____

Other:

_____   _____

It is also important to assess how effective your coping techniques are for dealing with drug issues. In the next section, begin by writing all of the coping mechanisms that you just listed in the first column under coping skills. Then in the next column, write how effective you feel this mechanism is in dealing with drug issues. Use a 0 to 10 scale (0 means totally useless in dealing with drug issues and 10 means totally effective). In the next column, place the word "yes" if you think the rating is adequate to deal with drug issues or "no" if you think it is not. Finally, in the last column, for those coping mechanisms that you felt were not adequate, try to suggest a different way to deal with drug issues that would make this technique more effective or that could be used instead of the technique that you see as ineffective.

Coping Skill	Effectiveness of the Skill in Dealing with Drug Issues (0–10)	Is This an Adequate Effectiveness Rating? (Yes/No)	Alternative Coping Skills to Deal with Drug Issues
_____	_____	_____	_____
_____	_____	_____	_____
_____	_____	_____	_____
_____	_____	_____	_____
_____	_____	_____	_____
_____	_____	_____	_____
_____	_____	_____	_____
_____	_____	_____	_____
_____	_____	_____	_____
_____	_____	_____	_____
_____	_____	_____	_____

A Good Offense: Drug Effects and Drug Substitutes

Drugs are used by athletes because they believe (rightly or wrongly) that certain effects will occur. It also has been said that there are no effects from drugs used in sports that cannot be achieved by an alternative, safer (and maybe even more effective) method. Therefore, a rational and independent approach to decisions about using drugs for sports involves asking yourself why you want to use a drug, what you hope to achieve, what the evidence is that the effects you seek will happen to you, and what the dangers are in using the drug. Perhaps more important, alternatives to using the drug, which also can achieve the desired effect, should be explored.

Completing the following chart for the Drug Options Plan and Evaluation (DOPE) for any drug that you think *might* have a place in sports can be helpful in organizing your thinking and making your decision.

Drug Options Plan and Evaluation

(DOPE)

Drug	Why Use— Expected Effects	Evidence to Support Desired Effects	Potential Dangers	Alternative Techniques for Same Effect/Result
___	___	___	___	___
___	___	___	___	___
___	___	___	___	___
___	___	___	___	___
___	___	___	___	___
___	___	___	___	___
___	___	___	___	___
___	___	___	___	___
___	___	___	___	___
___	___	___	___	___
___	___	___	___	___

If you are having some difficulty in coming up with "alternative techniques" to achieve the same effects that drugs are supposed to give you, it may be that you need to expand your understanding of sports science and sports training techniques. Different training regimens and nutritional strategies can be very helpful in improving performance results.

Another very important area that you might not be familiar with, but which can have very profound effects on your performance in sports, is the science of sports psychology. This is a relatively new emphasis in American sports, but is being seen by many athletes as being increasingly important. There are many books available that discuss how sports psychology can improve your athletic performance.

The importance of sport psychology for the athlete has recently been summarized by Olympian Lyle Nelson:

> The following sentence is the most powerful, all encompassing affirmation I can make for sport psychology. Your mental approach to conditioning and competing [which is sport psychology] determines how much you learn from your participation, the amount of enjoyment you experience, the number of years you will maintain interest, and your place on the results page. All athletic consequences are highly dependent on mental attributes.[2]

While it will be important for you to read further about various training techniques and sports psychology, some examples of how these approaches can be used to provide the same effects as drug use are provided in Table 9-1.

If you are not familiar with sports psychology, it is very important that you become so. You will probably find that such knowledge adds an incredibly positive dimension to your sports experience.

TECHNIQUES	GOALS		
	Feeling Up	Increased Strength/ Endurance	
Attention Control Training			
Biofeedback			
Centering	X		
Concentration Skill Training			
Dissociation			
Imagery	X	X	
Music	X		
Nutrition		X	
Progressive Muscle Relaxation			
Selective Association	X		
Self-Talk	X	X	
Stimulus Cueing			
Training/Conditioning Programs		X	
Visuo-Motor Behavior Rehearsal	X		

Alternatives to drugs that can be used to enhance performance in sports

Table 9-1

	Improved Concentration	Greater Confidence	Relaxation Competition/ Stress Management	Reducing Pain
	X	X	X	
			X	X
	X	X	X	X
	X	X		
			X	X
		X	X	X
			X	
			X	X
			X	
		X	X	X
	X			
		X		
		X	X	

Winning the Big Ones: Temptation Situations

You know there is something special about "the real thing." You can plan your performance all you want (and it's important to do this). You can practice as much as you can stand and even more. You can train and go beyond. Yet, when you walk onto the field, court, deck, or apparatus, the real thing is slightly different. Good training tries to simulate the real situation as much as possible.

The same is true for dealing with drug issues in sport. Planning to say no is great. Actually doing it can be much more difficult. One way to help insure that you will follow through with your decision is to anticipate the situations where you will have to live up to your decision, stand your ground. Trying to anticipate the tough situations *and* what you will *say* and *do* in them can take you one step closer to success in the actual situation.

Five tough temptation situations for drug use in sport are presented below. If you are to remain independent in your decision about drug use in your sport, you need to handle each one in the right way. Try to imagine or visualize each situation as realistically as possible. Place it in your own setting and add whatever details and aspects are important to you. Then also think about, visualize, and write down in the other columns (a) what you would think or say to yourself in the situation to avoid drug use; (b) what you would say out loud to others in the situation to help you refrain from drug use; and (c) what you would do in the situation to stand by your independent decision.

Saying No to Drugs

Winning the Big Ones: Temptation Situations

Situation I: You have just taken first place and won the championship. You are at a victory party and everyone is excited, happy, and celebrating. Someone suggests to you that you try a hit of a drug to really celebrate your achievement. What could it hurt?

What I Will Think or Say to Myself in the Situation

_____

_____

_____

_____

_____

What I Would Say to Others in the Situation

_____

_____

_____

_____

_____

What Actions I Would Take in the Situation

_____

_____

_____

_____

_____

Situation II: You are about the enter a crucial competition. You are up against your prime rival and competitor. You get wind of the fact that your competitor is using a drug in the upcoming event to help him get an edge. Someone tells you that you better use the drug, too, or you are sure to lose.

What I Will Think or Say to Myself in the Situation

_____

_____

_____

_____

_____

What I Would Say to Others in the Situation

_____

_____

_____

_____

_____

What Actions I Would Take in the Situation

_____

_____

_____

_____

_____

Situation III: You have hurt your leg playing touch football over the weekend and now the important competition is here, but your leg still aches. You went to the team physician, who tells you it would be best to rest the leg further. He is unwilling to prescribe any pain medication to you. You think that taking some drugs this one time might help you over the hump and through the competitive event.

What I Will Think or Say to Myself in the Situation

_____

_____

_____

_____

_____

What I Would Say to Others in the Situation

_____

_____

_____

_____

_____

What Actions I Would Take in the Situation

_____

_____

_____

_____

_____

Situation IV: You are away at an invitational meet. You are bunking with athletes from other cities and other parts of the country. They are all talking about a new performance-enhancing drug that is supposed to be great. Someone has some samples of it, wants to pass it around, and offers it to you to try.

What I Will Think or Say to Myself in the Situation

_____

_____

_____

_____

_____

What I Would Say to Others in the Situation

_____

_____

_____

_____

_____

What Actions I Would Take in the Situation

_____

_____

_____

_____

_____

Saying No to Drugs

Situation V: Over the last couple of weeks, your performance is below what it usually is. You seem to be in a little bit of a slump. You figure you can wait it out, but the team championship is coming up next week. The team captain corners you and asks you to take a performance-enhancing drug, just this one time for the team's sake.

What I Will Think or Say to Myself in the Situation

_____

_____

_____

_____

_____

What I Would Say to Others in the Situation

_____

_____

_____

_____

_____

What Actions I Would Take in the Situation

_____

_____

_____

_____

_____

After you have completed this exercise, you can visualize variations in these situations. Perhaps there are other situations that might be temptations for you, as well. Go through the same analyses as you just did with these five. Visualize and analyze the other situations. Best of all, get some teammates together and actually pretend that you are in the situation. Take turns playing different roles in each scene. Actually having performed the behavior—actually having thought, said, and done what you want to do—is much different and more effective than just planning to do it. Remember the lessons of real competition.

Chapter Ten

Prescribed Drugs in Sports:
THE ATHLETE WITH A MEDICAL CONDITION

Prescribed Drugs In Sports:
THE ATHLETE WITH A MEDICAL CONDITION

It is now clear that having a chronic medical condition is not a reason to avoid sports. Many individuals with a variety of medical problems compete and they do so seriously at all levels. Care for a medical condition may well involve the use of prescribed medications for cure, or for maintaining an optimal level of functioning.

While instructions from your doctor should always be followed in regard to such medication, there is a potential problem for competing athletes with a medical condition. If you have read this book carefully, you may have made certain observations about banned or illegal drugs from the sports perspective, as defined by the United States Olympic Committee, the International Olympic Committee, and the NCAA.

First, not all banned substances are so-called street or illegal drugs. Many drugs with important medical uses are banned because of abuse potential and/or unfair advantage in competition. Second, banned substances may be contained in various compounds so a banned drug might be taken inadvertently. None the less, this can lead to disqualification at levels where drug testing is enforced. Finally, IOC urine tests are qualitative only (for the presence of the drug). They are not quantitative; that is, they do not differentiate therapeutic or medically prescribed levels from abuse levels. Therefore, disqualification can occur even if a drug is taken only as prescribed and is not being abused (as has occurred).

So what should you do if you are an athlete who takes regular medication, but there is a chance that such use might create problems in terms of qualifying for a competition. There are several steps to consider (see Table 10-1).

First, *DO NOT* stop taking your medication. It has been given to you for a reason and you should continue to use it as directed. What you can and should do consists of the following steps:

1 *Contact your doctor.* You need to talk with your physician about what to do. If you have not in the past, you should certainly make sure that your doctor knows you are a competing athlete so that he may consider this when prescribing medication for you.

2 *In consultation with your doctor, check to see if any of the substances in your medication are prohibited.* Your doctor is the best person to know exactly what is contained in your medication. He is the one who can give you an expert opinion, which is preferable to your trying to determine this yourself.

3 *In consultation with your physician, discuss modification of your medication schedule.* In talking with your physician, you might be able to discuss other ways of taking your medication. Perhaps you can stop several days before a major competition. If this is not possible, your doctor may be able to switch you to a similar medication, one that can achieve the same results for your health, but that is not prohibited.

4 *Consider a medical declaration of need.* You and your physician together should investigate the drug abuse or drug testing rules and criteria for your particular sport as defined by its governing body. Generally there is a mechanism to allow athletes who are taking medication for their health to compete even though they are using the drug. Your doctor will have to fill out a Declaration of Need form or medical declaration. While such forms may vary, they usually required such information as a description of the

Prescribed Drugs in Sports

1 Do not stop taking your medication without your doctor's okay.

2 With your doctor, check to see if any ingredients in your medication are banned by your sport.

If banned substances are part of your medicine:

3 With your doctor, see if your medication schedule can be rearranged to avoid breaking the rules of your sport.

4 Have your doctor fill out the proper papers that might allow you to compete while taking your medicine. Complete a medical "Declaration of Need."

5 Request further information from the United States Olympic Committee at 1-800-233-0393.

Guidelines for Competing Athletes Using Medication to Treat a Medical Problem

Table 10-1

medical condition and the drug is needed; what drugs are actually being used (both the generic and trade names), and the like. This form is usually then presented to the medical director or person in charge of the meet or competition.

5 *When in doubt, contact the United States Olympic Committee.* The USOC supports a hotline for information about potentially banned or problematic drugs and medications. Whenever you have a question or concern, you can always contact the USOC for further information and direction. The hotline number for such questions and information is **1-800-233-0393.**

Prescribed Drugs in Sports

Chapter Eleven

Some Final Words:
TAKE IT FROM THEM

Some Final Words:
TAKE IT FROM THEM

This last section is a special one. In it you will find personal views about drugs and sports from those closest to sports and athletes. You will find comments from athletes themselves. There are thoughts from those who work with athletes. There are comments from sport psychologists who research and train athletes to apply techniques of performance enhancement and study the psychological health of athletes. If you are still unconvinced about the negative influence of drugs on sports and athletes, don't take it from me; take it from them.

Wayne "Tree" Rollins
Captain, Atlanta Hawks

I wish I had the right words to really explain how bad drugs are. I can try, but there always will be someone who won't get the message. Learning the lesson about drugs is more dangerous than learning about anything else. Learning the hard way about what drugs can do can mean death.

We know that drugs are powerful. We have seen what they can do to an athlete. But what people don't seem to realize is that drugs and drug use are very cunning and very deceptive. So many people have said, "It can't happen to me." Len Bias probably thought that. So did Don Rogers. Let me tell you, friends, that it CAN happen to you. Just like it happened to

Bias and Rogers in the prime of two magnificent athletic careers.

It's the drug that makes you think, "It can't happen to me." That's the deceptive part of drug use. You might have heard some of the other cunning phrases that drug users employ, too. "Just this once," "It's for fun," and "My friends are doing it and they seem to be OK," are just several of the lines that drugs use to attack and eventually ruin young people and young athletes.

I've never even tried drugs. But I have seen, with my own eyes, what they can do to an athlete. I have seen gifted athletes, people who were blessed by God with skills that I could only wish to have, lose those skills from the effects of drug use. I've seen people throw away everything that professional sports can provide—financial security, public acclaim, a glamorous life—because they made the mistake of trying a drug for the first time.

Those missed chances are just the side effects of what drugs can do. There's also the direct effect of drugs on the body of an athlete. Not everybody will become a professional athlete, but the effects are the same. The reactions needed for playing sports get dulled. The speed goes. So does the quickness. And so does the mind. The ability to concentrate, to think quickly, to visualize concepts—all become eroded by the use of drugs. I've seen the personality changes that come from drug use. Athletes who were once outgoing become withdrawn and paranoid. Players who were once confident become afraid of tasks that they once did instinctively. People who were once great unselfish teammates, who were fun to be with, get selfish on the court and go their own way off the court—off in search of that next, possibly fatal, hit; with so-called "friends" who don't care about team success, or the success of the player.

You might think I'm preaching. I am. In 10 years as a professional athlete I have seen what drugs can do to an athlete. Great players become nothing. Players with great potential never get the chance to achieve that potential. Yes, I'm preaching and I'll tell you why: You don't have to get an "F" on a test in school to know that you should have studied for the test beforehand. And you don't have to have your life ruined by drugs to know that you should have avoided them beforehand, either. If, as they say, experience is the best teacher, let the tragic experiences of Len Bias and Don Rogers be your teacher. Don't add your name to that list.

There are a number of ways that you can deal with this problem of drugs in your life. You can educate yourself about what they can do. You can remember the wasted potential of young athletes who never got the chance. You can think about how great Len Bias and Don Rogers were and what they are now. Or you can do the easiest and most effective thing of all: JUST SAY NO! I have. And it's worked great for me.

Athletes and Drugs

Dr. David A. Feigley
Director, Youth Sports Research Council
Rutgers University
New Brunswick, New Jersey

Gymnastics School Director
Gymnastics Coach
Former Competitive Diver

Perhaps the thing I value most in life is my independence and my ability to be in control of my life. Drugs are, in my opinion, the number one influence which could undermine that independence.

If you value your independence and truly want to control your own life, then you often have to make hard decisions. Being independent doesn't mean doing the opposite of what others advise you to do. Being contrary just means you are controlled in a different way. True independence, to me, means keeping control. Independent thinkers don't wear that independence on their sleeves or advertise it by their hair styles. They show it through their actions, which are often very quiet and unnoticed except by those around them who care enough to observe.

Drugs are one of life's true tests of independence. They are not the only serious test of independence but they are certainly a major one. Either you control your life or drugs do. That control is not "all or none" as some would suggest. But every time you "do drugs" you give up more control. The point at which you lose control is difficult to determine because drugs fool you! They give the illusion of giving you more control while they steal that control from you right before your very eyes.

People who say that experimenting with drugs will kill you are probably wrong. Statistics say that two people die from using cocaine every day. In a country of 226 million, that's not very frightening to me. However, losing control of my future does frighten me. I see addicts whose lives are wasted and who cause unbelievable long-term suffering and disappointment to those who love them. That to me is a true loss of control. Because of his sudden and unexpected death from cocaine, Len Bias doesn't know the suffering he caused those who loved him. He's dead. Drug addicts know what they are doing to themselves and to others who are important to them. They do it anyhow.

One reason I avoid drugs is because if others who look up to athletes and coaches see me do it, their chances of doing drugs goes up dramatically. As an athlete, look around you. All those youngsters who see you as a hero in sports are likely to try to copy you in other areas of their lives besides sport. You can choose to say that is not your responsibility, but such modeling occurs nonetheless. For my part, I refuse to be part of their problem.

If you think of yourself as a "clutch player" or if you want to be that person who "handles the big one," then deal with one of life's big ones. Peak performances require sacrifice. Only a few answer that challenge. When you see others doing drugs, you can rationalize that that makes it all right. After all, athletes are just like everyone else, aren't they? If you choose such a copout, that's your business. But don't for a minute believe that you are in control of your life or that you are that clutch player you might think you are. Drugs steal from you by making life appear easier than it truly is. Drugs give you a "certificate of participation" award. If you want the pride of real accomplishment, you will have to do it without drugs. Make your own choice!

DRUG ABUSE IN SPORT
based on an interview with
Scott McGregor,
Major League Pitcher

Until recently, I think most athletes were very unaware of the problem of drug abuse in sport. However, now many athletes are joining together to help fight drug abuse.

There are many reasons why athletes become involved in drug abuse. I think that perhaps the two most important ones are an abundance of money and idle time. These two elements spell trouble for anyone. This is especially true for young adult males.

Athletes use drugs for some of the same reasons as the general population, but also for different reasons. I think that stress is another main reason for drug abuse in our country in general, and stress is prevalent throughout our society as well as in sports.

Although many athletes hope to gain an edge, I don't believe that the use of drugs can improve athletic performance. Drug use may deceive you into thinking so, but drug abuse is a slow destruction of all motor skills. In fact, drugs may impair you because they throw off your system and destroy your skills. Athletics demand split-second decision making and you must have a clear mind to accomplish this.

I believe it is important for athletes to avoid the use of drugs for several reasons. First, all of us, but especially at the professional level, are role models to children and all of society. Second, drugs will end your career. Third, drugs will destroy your family or personal life.

I think there are several ways that athletes can say no to drugs. It is important to associate with the right crowd and stay away from the ones who are involved with drugs. Communicating with others who can help you if you are having trouble is very important; don't be a loner. Idle time also brings many temptations. Along with this, I have found that having a purpose in my life is very important. For me, it is my faith in God. If you don't have vision in your life, you won't accomplish anything. The proper motivation is essential. If money and fame are your only criteria, you will always be frustrated.

In short, I think that drug abuse has tarnished the image of sports and athletes. We are very visible and very influential.

We are sending out the wrong message to America. Tearing off the tops of beer cans and abusing cocaine don't help build a strong society. As an athlete, if you feel that you have a drug problem, go talk to those who can help. This means your team physicians, family, or clergy. When you are in this situation, you must confront the problem and set a course to flee from it.

The Impact of Drugs on Sports and Athletics

by Shane M. Murphy, Ph.D.
Head, Department of Sport Psychology
Sports Science Program
United States Olympic Committee
Colorado Springs, Colorado

When I was asked to think about the subject of drugs in sports, two major issues came to my mind. One is the problems that using so-called recreational drugs can cause for athletes. The other issue is the misuse of ergogenic aids, such as steroids, by athletes trying to improve their performance.

I will talk about the ergogenic aids issue first. There is no doubt that this problem worries many athletes I speak to, especially in some sports where there is a widespread perception that you have to use drugs to keep up with the competition. But we have to be careful that we don't rely on this issue as a crutch or an excuse. I have visited many countries and spoken to athletes from all over the world, and I know that all of us sometimes make the mistake of assuming that this problem exists when it doesn't. Many of us here in the United States, for example, point to eastern European countries and say that a lot of their athletic performances are helped by use of various ergogenic drugs. But if you talk to eastern European athletes and other foreign competitors, many are convinced that US athletes have attained superiority through the use of ergogenic aids! I know about two cases this year where US athletes won international competitions, and other countries pointed at us and said "drugs." But those athletes were drug-free! We undoubtedly make the same mistake if we glibly attribute foreign triumphs to drug-related enhancement. In our Sports Science Department at the USOC, we often find that world champions in various sports have a clear edge over their competitors in technique or in training methods. As athletes and coaches, we make it too easy for ourselves to begin using questionable methods, such as using drugs, if we assume that "everyone else is doing it" when we don't know the facts.

One development that encourages me is that some sports have really made a big effort lately to help their young athletes stay drug-free. And it's working! The sports are helping coaches and athletes develop that "extra edge" by developing new training programs; understanding the latest developments in physiology, such as periodized training; getting expert help, such as from biomechanists, in developing technique and learning new skills; and working on mental training programs. With all those added advantages to traditional training, there is no need to go searching for some "magic pill" that may cause very serious long-term damage to the athlete. It's too risky.

I will be brief in my comments about the second issue. I have not seen many problems with "recreational" drug abuse in amateur athletics, except for some alcohol abuse. That may be because these drugs interfere with performance—you can't keep taking them without people noticing deterioration in your performance. And most amateur athletes are not wealthy. Drugs like cocaine cost a lot of money. But if an athlete does develop a drug abuse problem, the reasons are usually the same as those of a nonathlete. The drug is being used to fill some gap, some void, in the person's life. The athlete can be helped by seeing a drug abuse counselor, who will help develop a program to control and eliminate drug abuse, and help identify what gap lead to the drug use initially.

Why Should I Say No?

Josie Todd
Women's Varsity Basketball
University of Illinois at Urbana-Champaign

As an athlete you are a special person. You are unique because in addition to your regular responsibilities you have chosen to challenge yourself in sports. By accepting this challenge you have also accepted the responsibilities that accompany sports participation. With this in mind, you must consider the issue of drug and alcohol use.

Like other individuals, athletes like yourself will have many choices to make in life, and one of the most important choices will focus on whether to use drugs and alcohol. Looking back on my high school days, I remember my coach saying, 'stay away from drugs,' and most of my teammates did. Some of my friends, however, when faced with the decision to use drugs, often thought to themselves, "why should I say no?"

For the athlete who wants to be the best he or she can be, the answer to the question "why say no" is that drugs hurt athletic performance. And because drugs hinder and prevent optimal performance, they have no value to the dedicated athlete. They are defeating to the body, and it makes no sense to work and train on developing your body just to hurt it by abusing drugs.

In addition to realizing that drugs hurt performance, you must also remember your responsibility to the team, the school, and the spectators who encourage you in athletics. You are not just another person, but one of the most visible individuals in your community. Because of this, you assume the responsibility of serving as a role model, especially for those younger athletes in the community. In essence, by accepting the challenge of sports you must realize that you have an impact on your friends and the spectators who watch you. Moreover, because your actions set a precedent for others, they not only affect you, but a number of other individuals who look to you for leadership. Hence, any decision to engage in alcohol and drugs is more than a personal decision.

There is another more basic reason why you should say no to drugs. Simply put, it is illegal for high school athletes to use alcohol and for athletes of any age to use drugs. And this, more than any other reason, should make an athlete think again before using drugs. The penalties for being caught with drugs are stiff, and to the athlete who loves his or her sport, the risk of getting caught is just too great. The threat of being kicked off the team, in addition to any penalties dictated by law, are just too severe for the dedicated athlete to even consider using drugs.

Drugs are illegal; they hinder athletic performance; and drugs have no place in the life of an athlete who is a role model. So why do athletes use drugs? Some do it to fit in; some do it "for the thrills"; others do it to relieve stress. The athletes who truly love sports and the competition they face say "no" because they won't let anything get in the way of their goals. As an athlete you are special, but the choice is the same. "Should I or shouldn't I try drugs?" And this is no easy choice, as one of the most difficult things to do is to say "no" to drugs in the presence of friends. But it is also not easy to make the team, sink that critical free-throw at the end of the game, or push yourself to the limits in the weight room. The challenge I pose to you is to dare to be special, dare to say "no" to drugs, and dare to be great.

You And Substance Abuse: Think Before You Leap!

**Daniel Gould, PhD, Associate Professor
Co-Editor, *The Sport Psychologist*
University of North Carolina at
Greensboro
Department of Physical Education**

Sharon has lung cancer, is bald from chemotherapy treatments and has been given six months to live. She began smoking as a collegiate golfer. She really disliked the taste of smoke when she started, but wanted to fit in with her roommates who all smoked. After college she tried to kick the habit several times, but just could not do it. She was hooked.

Ronnie graduated from college five years ago. As a small tight end he took steroids in an effort to bulk up for the pros.

He was able to gain 30 pounds, but was not drafted. The pro scouts said he had poor hands and was unable to run precise pass routes. Ronnie is now back to his normal weight of 195 pounds, but has been in and out of the hospital with liver and kidney problems. Oh yes, Ronnie and his wife Shanda recently learned that they cannot have children because Ronnie is sterile—another side effect of his past steroid use.

Jim was looking forward to his senior year on the Miller High basketball team. He was the starting point guard on a team of five returning starters who finished second in the state last year. Unfortunately, Jim won't be playing the rest of the season. He was dismissed from the team when he was picked up for driving while intoxicated on his way home from a post-game party after the team's first victory of the young season.

Finally, Sandy just cannot seem to cope with the pressure. Her parents expect all A's in school, her teachers constantly talk about her as a model student, implying that she should be perfect at everything she does, and her teammates always count on her in the clutch. Sandy's found that smoking a joint and popping an array of uppers relieves the stress. As of late, however, she has found that she needs a fix more frequently and always before games or tests.

All four of these scenarios depict negative side effects of alcohol and drug abuse. However, they also reflect several important psychological issues that should be considered before anyone uses alcohol or drugs.

The first important issue to consider is that none of these individuals made a well-thought out decision to utilize these substances. Sharon smoked because her roommates did. Ronnie took steroids thinking it was the magic pill that would take him to the pros, Jim was out celebrating the first win of the season, and Sandy was just trying to cope. Unfortunately, none of these athletes realized the long-term ramifications of their decisions until it was too late.

What about you? Have you stopped to think about the short and long-term ramifications of such decisions? Or will you get sucked into doing what everyone else does? Take a few minutes right now to list the pros and cons of such decisions, when there is time to think about things and no pressure to act from others. In essence, take the time to think before you leap! Moreover, if you do not know the actual facts about alcohol and drug use go to your school library and read about the issue or watch a video on the subject.

A second important consideration reflected in the examples above is that at times athletes look for unrealistic and easy solutions to complex problems. This is not uncommon or unique to these individuals—we all do it. For example, as a sport psychology consultant, I am frequently asked by athletes and coaches to identify easy solutions, quick fixes or miracle cures which will suddenly mentally and emotionally prepare them for competition. After all, they know I am an expert in the area so I must know the secrets of success. It is unfortunate that I and other sport psychologists do not have such simple fixes or magic cures. What we have learned through research and practice is that great athletes develop psychological skills much like they learn physical skills, through good instruction, hard work, discipline and practice. It is the same with using drugs and alcohol to solve problems. Taking pills did not help Sandy cope with the pressure in the long run. It only made her dependent on the pills. She would have been much better off learning and practicing the stress management techniques sport psychologists are using to help Olympic and Professional athletes. Similarly, the steroids did not guarantee Ronnie a pro career or even a tryout. He needed to work on skill development, and perhaps, set more realistic goals.

In summary, when you're faced with a tough problem do not expect easy answers or magic cures. If an athlete wants to overcome complex problems he or she must learn as much as possible about the problem, develop long-term plans, get help from knowledgable others and work very hard.

What about you? Do you have problems coping with pressure, being accepted by your friends or achieving your goals? If the answer to any of these questions is yes, don't panic. Think before you leap for a miracle cure in a bottle or pill. Learn more about the problem, types of strategies available to solve it, and who is available and knowledgeable to help you work through it. These problems are not unique and have been faced by others. More importantly, they can all be solved, but you must be realistic in your approach and develop a well thought out game plan for solving them.

In conclusion, most athletes who have problems with substance abuse did not consider the long-term ramifications of their initial involvement with the substance. They used these substances in an effort to fit in, in efforts to cope with immediate problems, or because everyone else used them. Unfortunately, by the time the ramifications were apparent it was too late to turn the clock back. A smart athlete learns from the mistakes of others on the field or in the gym. Be a smart athlete out of the arena or off the field and look before you leap and think before you act—especially when it comes to drug and alcohol use!

Drugs and Alcohol Use in High School Athletics

Thomas W. Bay
Certified Athletic Trainer
Central Dauphin High School
Harrisburg, PA

Is the use of drugs and alcohol prevalent among high school athletes? It is always hard to determine the exact percentage of such use by athletes. However, from previous surveys and reports done throughout school districts across the nation, it is obvious that athletes are not immune to the drug and alcohol problem.

It has been my experience that on the high school level, alcohol is probably more abused than other drugs. However, the drug situation cannot be overlooked because of the many different drugs and the many different ways they can affect an individual athlete. Some of the more common drugs which high school athletes come in contact with are marijuana, cocaine, amphetamines, and anabolic steroids.

How does one begin to find out about drug and alcohol use among athletes? Some programs have been very successful in conducting a survey which helps determine what drugs and alcohol are being used, how often they are being used, and why. More is needed than just this, however. The importance of having some type of drug and alcohol abuse prevention program for athletes in the high school environment is all too often overlooked.

The program should certainly be preventative in nature as well as informative. Some way for athletes who have problems to confidentially admit them and seek help is also highly desirable. The total commitment of school officials and community support is needed to help build a successful prevention program. Along with the coaches, parents, and community involvement, athletes must also work with their respective teammates to help any drug or alcohol related problem.

What happens if an athlete is suspected of drug or alcohol use? What actions should be implemented? I would make sure that adequate information is obtained, and then approach the athlete with the available information. Informing parents, coaches, or relevant school officials as necessary and as the situation warrants about the particular problem should also be considered.

In one case, I had involvement with an athlete who was taking an over-the-counter diet suppressant. After an interscholastic event, the athlete was taken to the hospital. During questioning about any medications, the athlete mentioned the diet suppressant. The athlete was then talked to confidentially by the coach, team physician and athletic trainer. The parent was also informed of the situation. It can be best to ask the athlete him or herself to do the informing of the parents, but care must be taken that this actually does occur. Impressed upon the athlete were some of the drastic results that could potentially happen physically, as well as the athlete's probable discontinuation in scholastic sport should the problem ever surface again.

Hopefully successful drug abuse prevention programs will minimize the need for unpleasant situations just described. I certainly feel every school district should have at least some type of program implemented to meet the needs of any drug or alcohol related problem among its athletes. High school is a critical training ground for future levels of athletic performance and physical and psychological health for the athlete.

Athletes in high school are under great peer pressure, and they need to know the impact that drugs or alcohol can have on them now and later in life. They also need a way to seek help for their problem while feeling supported and safe rather than threatened in doing so.

FOOTNOTES

Introduction

1. ————, "Drug Abuse in Sports: Denial Fuels the Problem," *The Physician and Sportsmedicine,* 1982, *10*(4): 114.

2. Adapted from *The Physician and Sportsmedicine,* 1982, *10*(4): 122.

3. R. Reilly, "When the Cheers Turned to Tears," *Sports Illustrated,* 14 July 1986, 29.

Chapter 2

1. The pronoun "he" is used for editorial convenience only. Comments apply to female athletes as well, and the term "he" is not used to ignore or be disrespectful of female athletes.

Chapter 6

1. ————, "Drug Abuse in Sports: Denial Fuels the Problem," *The Physician and Sportsmedicine,* 1982, *10*(4): 118.

2. Ibid.

Chapter 7

1. T. Murray, "The Coercive Power of Drugs in Sport,' *The Hastings Center Report,* August 1983: 27.

2. T. Murray, "Get on with Sports, Leave Steroids Behind," *The Physician and Sportsmedicine,* 1984, *12*(3): 187.

3. Ibid.

4. Quoted in "Drug Abuse in Sports: Denial Fuels the Problem," *The Physician and Sportsmedicine,* 1982, *10*(4): 123.

Chapter 8

1. The regulatory status of various drugs is generally changing because of review and decision processes. The regulatory status described here for various drugs is a guideline only. Exact and current status information should be obtained as needed from the appropriate governing organization.

2. ———, "Drug Abuse in Sports: Denial Fuels the Problem," *The Physician and Sportsmedicine,* 1982, *10*(4): 119.

3. R. Reilly, "When the Cheers Turn to Tears," *Sports Illustrated,* 14 July 1986, 30.

4. E. Percy, "Chemical Warfare: Drugs in Sports," *The Western Journal of Medicine,* 1980, 133: 480.

Chapter 9

1. L. Nelson, "The Athlete's Perspective" in J. May and M. Asken (eds.), *Sport Psychology: The Psychological Health of the Athlete* (Great Neck, N.Y.: PMA Publishers, 1987), 261.

2. Ibid., 256.

REFERENCES

———— (1982). Drug abuse in sports: Denial fuels the problem. *The Physician and Sportsmedicine, 10* (4): 114–23.

———— (1986). Crack, *The Medical Letter, 28* (718): 69–70.

American College of Sports Medicine (1978). Position statement on the use and abuse of anabolic-androgenic steroids in sports. *The Physician and Sportsmedicine, 6* (3):157–58.

American College of Sports Medicine (1982). Position statement on the use of alcohol in sports. *Medicine and Science in Sports and Exercise, 14* (6): ix–xi.

American College of Sports Medicine (1987). Position statement on the use of anabolic-androgenic steroids in sports. *Medicine and Science in Sports and Exercise, 19* (5): 534–39.

American College of Sports Medicine (1987). Position statement on blood doping as an ergogenic aid. *Medicine and Science in Sports and Exercise, 19* (5): 540–43.

Asken, M. (1985). Sport psychology and high school coaches: A survey. *Pennsylvania Journal of Health, Physical Education, Recreation and Dance, 55* (2): 4–6.

Blum, K. (1984). *Handbook of Abusable Drugs.* New York: Gardiner Press, Inc.

Chappel, J. (1987). Drug Use and Abuse in the Athletes. In J. May & M. Asken (eds.) *Sport Psychology: The Psychological Health of the Athlete.* Great Neck, N.Y.: PMA Publishers.

Clement, D. (1983). Drug use survey: Result and conclusion. *The Physician and Sportsmedicine, 11* (9): 64–67.

Cohen, S. (1969). *The Drug Dilemma.* New York: McGraw-Hill.

Cohen, S. (1981). *The Substance Abuse Problems: Volume I.* New York: The Haworth Press.

Cohen, S. (1985). *The Substance Abuse Problems: Volume II: New Issues for the 1980's.* New York: The Haworth Press.

Collins, G., Pippenger, C., and Janesz, J. (1984). Links in the chain: An approach to the treatment of drug abuse on a professional football team. *Cleveland Clinic Quarterly, 51:* 485–92.

Crawshaw, J. (1985). Recognizing anabolic steroid abuse. *Patient Care, 19:* 28–47.

Dardik, I. (1984). Breaking the 'Breakthrough myth.' *The Physician and Sportsmedicine, 12* (3): 183.

Demak, R. (1986). And then she just disappeared. *Sports Illustrated,* June 16: 18.

Dintimen, G., and Unitas, J. (1979). *Improving Health and Performance in the Athlete.* Englewood Cliffs, N.J.: Prentice-Hall.

Dolan, E. (1986). *Drugs in Sport.* New York: Franklin Watts.

Dyment, P. (1982). Drug misuse by adolescent athletes. *Pediatric Clinics of North America, 29* (6): 1363–68.

Eck, W. (1982). Strategy for implementation of an alcohol education program. *Journal of Drug Education, 12* (4): 285–87.

Gardiner, P. (1983). Anti-inflammatory medications. *The Physician and Sportsmedicine, 11* (9): 71–73.

Garfield, E., and Jones, D. (1980). Drug education group process: Considerations for the classroom. *Journal of Drug Education, 10* (2): 101–109.

Gilman, A., Goodman, L., Rall, T., and Murad, F. (1985). *Goodman and Gilman's The Pharmacological Basis of Therapeutics. (7th Ed.).* New York: Macmillan Publishing Company.

Goodstadt, M. (1980). Drug education—a turn on or turn off? *Journal of Drug Education, 10* (2): 89–99.

Griffin, T. (1985). *Paying the Price.* Center City, Minn.: The Hazeldon Foundation.

Hatfield, B., and Sullivan, K. (1987). The business of sport and the athlete. In J. May & M. Asken (eds.) *Sport Psychology: The Psychological Health of the Athlete.* Great Neck, N.Y.: PMA Publishers.

Haupt, H., and Rovere, G. (1984). Anabolic steroids: A review of the literature. *The American Journal of Sports Medicine, 12* (6): 469–84.

Herbert, V. (1979). Pangamic Acid ("Vitamin B$_{15}$") *The American Journal of Clinical Nutrition, 37:* 1534–40.

Hill-Donisch, K., Orange, C., and Webster, T. (1987). *Women in Sports and Chemical Use: Breaking the Silence.* Minneapolis, Minn.: Hazeldon-Cork Sports Education Program.

Johanson, C. (1986). *Cocaine: A New Epidemic.* New York: Chelsea House Publishers.

Kimiecik, J. (1987). Coaches go to class for drug education. *American Coach,* Sept.–Oct: 1.

Kulund, D. (1982). *The Injured Athlete.* Philadelphia: J. B. Lippincott.

Laties, V., and Weiss, B. (1981). The amphetamine margin in sports. *Federation Proceedings, 40:* 2689–92.

Legwold, G. (1984). Have we learned a lesson about drugs in sports? *The Physician and Sportsmedicine, 12* (3): 175–80.

Lukas, S. (1985). *Amphetamines: Danger in the Fast Lane.* New York: Chelsea House Publishers.

MacDougall, D. (1983). Anabolic steroids. *The Physician and Sportsmedicine, 11* (9): 95–101.

Martz, L., Millwe, M., Cohn, B., Raine, G., and Carroll, G. (1986). Trying to say "No". *Newsweek,* August 11: 14–15.

McCallum, J. (1986), The cruelest thing ever, *Sports Illustrated,* June 30: 20–27.

McEvoy, G. (ed.) *AHTS Drug Information 1987.* Bethesda, Md.: American Society of Hospital Pharmacists.

Murray, T. (1983). The coercive power of drugs in sports. *The Hastings Center Report,* August: 24–30.

Murray, T. (1984). Get on with sports, leave steroids behind. *The Physician and Sportsmedicine, 12* (3): 187.

Nelson, L. (1987). The athlete's perspective. In J. May & M. Asken (eds.) *Sport Psychology: The Psychological Health of the Athlete.* Great Neck, N.Y.: PMA Publishers.

Oseid, S. (1984). Doping and athletes: Prevention and counseling. *Journal of Allergy and Clinical Immunology, 73:* 735–39.

Percy, E. (1980). Chemical warfare. Drugs in sports. *Western Journal of Medicine, 133:* 478–84.

Prokop, L. (1975). Drug abuse in international athletics. *Journal of Sports Medicine, 3* (2): 85–87.

Puffer, J. (1986). The use of drugs in swimming. *Clinics in Sports Medicine, 5* (1): 77–89.

Randall, D., and Wong, M. (1976). Drug education to date: A review. *Journal of Drug Education, 6* (1): 1–21.

Reilly, R. (1986). When the cheers turned to tears. *Sports Illustrated,* July 14: 28–34.

Ryan, A. (1981). Anabolic steroids are fool's gold. *Federation Proceedings, 49* (12): 2682–88.

Ryan, A. (1984). Causes and remedies for drug misuse and abuse by athletes. *Journal of the American Medical Association, 252* (4): 517–19.

Scott, W., Nisonson, B., and Nicholas, J. (eds.) (1984). *Principles of Sports Medicine,* Baltimore: Williams and Wilkins.

Shear, M. (1987). The smokeless scandal. *The Main Event: Monthly Sports Journal for Physicians, 2* (11): 30–31.

Sheppard, M. (1983). Development of a cannabis education program. *Journal of Drug Education, 13* (2): 115–17.

Smith, G. (1983). Recreational drugs in sports. *The Physician and Sports-medicine, 11* (9): 75–82.

Strauss, R. (ed.) (1987). *Drugs and Performance in Sport.* Philadelphia: W. B. Saunders.

Svendsen, R., Griffin, T., and McIntyre, D. (1984). *Chemical Health: School Athletics and Fine Art Activities.* Center City, Minn.: Hazelden Foundation.

US Department of Justice, Drug Enforcement Agency (1984). *Team Up for Drug Prevention.* Washington, D.C.: U.S. Government Printing Office. Publication #0-459-002.

US Department of Justice, Drug Enforcement Agency (1986). *For Coaches Only: How to Start a Drug Prevention Program.* Washington, D.C.: U.S. Government Printing Office. Publication #0-167-916 (QL-3).

United States Olympic Committee (1986). *US Olympic Committee Drug Control Program Protocol 1985–88.* Colorado Springs, Colo.: US Olympic Committee.

United States Olympic Committee (1987). *Drug Education Newsletter, 1* (2): 1–4.

United States Olympic Committee, Committee on Substance Abuse Research and Education (1987). *USOC Drug Control Program: Questions and Answers.* Colorado Springs, Colo.: US Olympic Committee.

Webb, R., Egger, G., and Reynolds, I. (1978). Prediction and prevention of drug abuse. *Journal of Drug Education, 8* (3): 221–29.

Zoller, W., and Weiss, S. (1981). "Hashish & Marijuana" An innovative, interdisciplinary drug education curricular program for high schools. *Journal of Drug Education, 11* (1): 37–46.

About the Author

Michael Asken, Ph.D., completed his undergraduate education at the Johns Hopkins University where he graduated with honors. He received his master's and doctoral degrees from West Virginia University in clinical psychology with a minor in medical psychology.

Dr. Asken is currently in the private practice of clinical/health psychology and sport psychology consultation with Cowley Associates Medical Group in Camp Hill, Pennsylvania. Prior to this, he was associate director for preventive medicine and health psychology in the Department of Family Medicine at Polyclinic Medical Center in Harrisburg, Pennsylvania. He is an adjunct assistant professor of behavioral sciences at the Pennsylvania State University College of Medicine, M.S. Hershey Medical Center. As an adjunct associate professor of psychology at Lebanon Valley College, he teaches sport psychology.

Dr. Asken is a fellow and a diplomat of the American Board of Medical Psychotherapists. He is a member of the American Psychological Association, the Society of Behavioral Medicine, and Academy of Psychosomatic Medicine, and a fellow of the Pennsylvania Psychological Association.

In relation to sport psychology, Dr. Asken is a member of the International Society of Sport Psychology and a charter member of the Association for the Advancement of Applied Sport Psychology. He is a committee chairperson for the Division of Exercise and Sport Psychology of the American Psychological Association, and a consultant in sport psychology to local sport organizations. He was co-chairman of the United States Olympic Committee's 1987 National Conference on Sport Psychology. He is co-editor of a recent book, *Sport Psychology: The Psychological Health of the Athlete.*